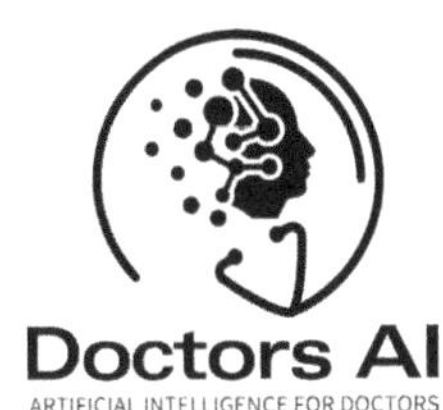

Decoding
Artificial Intelligence
for Physicians

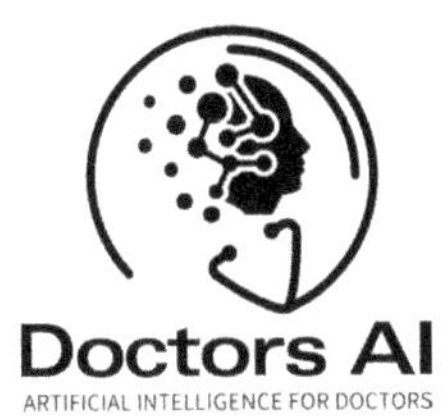

Decoding Artificial Intelligence
for Physicians

Shambo Samrat Samajdar

MBBS MD DM (Clinical Pharmacology), FIPS Fellow Diabetes India
PG Dip Endo & Diabetes (RCP)
Fellowship in Respiratory and Critical Care (WBUHS)
Diploma in Allergy Asthma Immunology (BV University)

Consultant, Diabetes and Allergy-Asthma Therapeutics Specialty Clinic
Kolkata, West Bengal, India
Research Wing Leader, Doctors AI

Amit Kumar Dey

MBBS MD FACP (USA), FRSPH (UK), FDI ABAIM (USA)
Dip. Geriatric Medicine, Dip. MSc (Diabetology) (UK)

Consultant: Diabetes, Obesity & Metabolic Disorders, Kolkata, West Bengal, India
Founder Chair: Doctors AI

Bharat Saboo

MBBS MSc Endocrinology, Diploma in Diabetology
Scope Certified (Obesity)

Director and Chief Consultant Diabetologist
Prayas Diabetes Center, Indore, Madhya Pradesh, India
Co-founder: Doctors AI

Forewords

◆ **Jyotirmoy Pal**   ◆ **Peter Schwarz**   ◆ **Shashank R Joshi**   ◆ **Banshi Saboo**   ◆ **Anuj Maheswari**

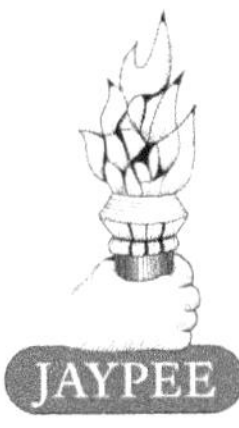

JAYPEE

JAYPEE BROTHERS MEDICAL PUBLISHERS
The Health Sciences Publisher
New Delhi | London

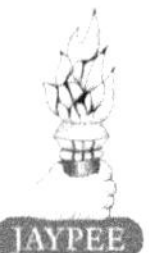 **Jaypee Brothers Medical Publishers (P) Ltd**

Headquarters
EMCA House
23/23-B, Ansari Road, Daryaganj
New Delhi 110 002, India
Landline: +91-11-23272143, +91-11-23272703
+91-11-23282021, +91-11-23245672
E-mail: jaypee@jaypeebrothers.com

Corporate Office
Jaypee Brothers Medical Publishers (P) Ltd.
4838/24, Ansari Road, Daryaganj
New Delhi 110 002, India
Phone: +91-11-43574357
Fax: +91-11-43574314
E-mail: jaypee@jaypeebrothers.com

Overseas Office
JP Medical Ltd.
83, Victoria Street, London
SW1H 0HW (UK)
Phone: +44-20 3170 8910
E-mail: info@jpmedpub.com

EU GPSR Authorised Representative
Logos Europe, 9 rue Nicolas Poussin
17000, La Rochelle, France
Phone: +33 (0) 6 67 93 73 78
E-mail: Contact@logoseurope.eu

Website: www.jaypeebrothers.com
Website: www.jaypeedigital.com

© 2025, Jaypee Brothers Medical Publishers

Inquiries for bulk sales may be solicited at: jaypee@jaypeebrothers.com

Decoding Artificial Intelligence for Physicians

First Edition: **2025**
ISBN: 978-93-6616-302-4

Dedication

This book is humbly dedicated to *Mahakal*, the timeless guardian of life and death, the embodiment of eternal truth, and the ultimate source of wisdom and compassion. In this journey of unraveling the mysteries of modern medicine through the lens of artificial intelligence, we seek the divine grace and guidance of Lord Mahakal, who transcends all boundaries of time, knowledge, and existence.

We invoke the power of the *Mahamrityunjaya Mantra*, a sacred prayer that bestows healing, vitality, and liberation:

ॐ त्र्यम्बकं यजामहे सुगन्धिं पुष्टिवर्धनम् |
उर्वारुकमिव बन्धनान्मृत्योर्मुक्षीय माऽमृतात् ||

"Om Tryambakam Yajamahe Sugandhim Pushtivardhanam|
Urvarukamiva Bandhanan Mrityor Mukshiya Maamritat||"

In these words, we seek protection from the cycle of suffering, guidance toward spiritual growth, and liberation from the bonds of mortality. May this sacred mantra inspire all who read this work to cultivate a spirit of compassion, humility, and dedication in their practice. May it remind us that every advancement in science and technology, every discovery in medicine, is merely a humble step on the path of serving humanity under the watchful grace of the Divine.

Foreword

It is a privilege to write the foreword for *Decoding Artificial Intelligence for Physicians*, a pioneering work that seeks to bridge the gap between advanced technology and clinical practice. This book arrives at a crucial juncture, where healthcare professionals are being called upon to integrate new technologies, such as artificial intelligence (AI), into their daily practice. As President-Elect of the Association of Physicians of India (API) and Past Dean of the Indian College of Physicians, I have observed firsthand the evolution of medical practice and the importance of staying abreast of technological advancements. This book, authored by Dr Shambo Samrat Samajdar, Dr Amit Kumar Dey, and Dr Bharat Saboo, serves as a comprehensive guide to understanding and applying AI in a clinical context.

Artificial intelligence has emerged as a transformative force in healthcare, capable of enhancing diagnostics, improving treatment plans, and streamlining workflows. This transformation is particularly significant in a country like India, where healthcare systems face challenges of scale, resource constraints, and a diverse patient's population. The authors of this book adeptly cover these aspects and more, providing a roadmap for clinicians who seek to harness AI to improve patient's care. Their work is enriched with practical case studies, theoretical insights, and assessments that cater to a range of readers, from postgraduate students to experienced medical practitioners.

One of the most impressive aspects of *Decoding Artificial Intelligence for Physicians* is its ability to take a complex and often intimidating topic and make it both comprehensible and practical. The book covers foundational AI concepts, such as machine learning and deep learning, and dives into their real-world applications across various specialties, including endocrinology, cardiology, neurology, and more. These chapters are thoughtfully structured, providing readers with both the theoretical knowledge and the clinical implications of AI.

As a Professor of Medicine in West Bengal, I have witnessed how the implementation of digital tools and AI-driven applications can drastically enhance the quality of care. From early disease detection and risk stratification to personalized medicine, AI offers solutions that were once beyond our reach. This book highlights how AI-driven technologies can optimize patient's management, monitor chronic conditions, and provide decision support, thus enabling physicians to make more informed and effective clinical decisions.

However, with great potential comes great responsibility. AI's integration into healthcare is not without its challenges. Issues related to data security, algorithmic fairness, and maintaining the ethical standards of medical practice are critical considerations that must not be overlooked. I commend the authors for their balanced approach, which includes discussions on regulatory frameworks, patient's consent, and the importance of human oversight. This ensures that physicians are not only equipped with the tools to adopt AI but also with the knowledge to implement it in an ethical and patient-centered manner.

The book's practical approach, including real-world case scenarios and comprehensive multiple-choice questions, makes it an invaluable resource for postgraduate students preparing for competitive examinations and for physicians who wish to deepen their understanding of AI applications in clinical practice. These features make the book a versatile guide that supports lifelong learning and the continuous development of medical expertise.

I believe that *Decoding Artificial Intelligence for Physicians* will inspire healthcare professionals to embrace AI thoughtfully and responsibly. It provides a clear vision of how technology can enhance patient's care without compromising the fundamental principles of medicine. The authors have done a commendable job of creating a resource that not only educates but also empowers, setting the stage for a future where AI and clinical practice coexist harmoniously for the benefit of patients.

In closing, I congratulate Dr Shambo Samrat Samajdar, Dr Amit Kumar Dey, and Dr Bharat Saboo for their significant contribution to medical literature. This book is a testament to their dedication and vision, and I am confident that it will serve as a guiding resource for physicians navigating the complex landscape of AI in healthcare.

Jyotirmoy Pal
MBBS MD (General Medicine) FRCP FICP FACP WHO Fellow
President-Elect, Association of Physicians of India (API)
Past Dean, Indian College of Physicians

Foreword

As we stand on the precipice of a new era in medical innovation, it is a privilege and an honor to contribute a foreword to *Decoding Artificial Intelligence for Physicians*, a comprehensive and timely work that underscores the transformative role of artificial intelligence (AI) in modern healthcare. This book arrives at a pivotal moment when medicine and technology converge to forge a path toward more personalized, predictive, and efficient patient's care.

In my role as the Head of the Division for Prevention and Care of Diabetes and President of the International Diabetes Federation (IDF), I have witnessed firsthand the potential of digital tools and AI to enhance the way we prevent and manage chronic diseases, particularly type 2 diabetes mellitus. My research, which spans molecular and clinical mechanisms, has consistently demonstrated that leveraging digital solutions, including AI-powered smartphone applications, can address common lifestyle-associated risk factors more effectively than traditional approaches alone.

What makes *Decoding Artificial Intelligence for Physicians* an essential read is its holistic and multispecialty approach. The authors—Dr Shambo Samrat Samajdar, Dr Amit Kumar Dey, and Dr Bharat Saboo—have skillfully compiled knowledge and practical applications that guide physicians through the integration of AI in various clinical settings. From enhancing diagnostic accuracy to supporting patient's adherence and education, this book navigates the complex terrain of AI with clarity and depth.

The chapters provide an invaluable resource not only for endocrinologists like myself but also for clinicians across specialties who are keen to understand how AI can be applied to improve patient's outcomes. The authors delve into real-world case studies that reflect the tangible benefits AI offers, while also addressing the challenges and ethical considerations that accompany its use. This balanced perspective ensures that the reader is equipped with both the theoretical foundations and the practical tools needed to harness AI's capabilities responsibly and effectively.

Artificial intelligence's promise in diabetes care, in particular, is profound. Tools that integrate AI-driven data analysis, lifestyle interventions, and personalized treatment plans are poised to revolutionize our approach to prevention and management. With AI, we can identify individuals at risk earlier, predict disease progression with greater accuracy, and develop tailored interventions that improve both patient's outcomes and quality of life.

However, as with any revolutionary tool, the implementation of AI in healthcare requires careful consideration of its limitations, ethical implications, and potential biases. The authors of this book do not shy away from these discussions; instead, they emphasize the importance of regulatory compliance, data integrity, and collaboration between AI developers and medical professionals to ensure that AI serves as a complement to, not a replacement for, human expertise.

As healthcare professionals, we must remain open to continuous learning and adaptation. *Decoding Artificial Intelligence for Physicians* not only prepares readers to understand and utilize current AI applications but also encourages them to anticipate future innovations. It is a work that bridges the gap between technological potential and clinical application, empowering physicians to lead the charge in integrating AI into their practice for the betterment of patient's care.

In closing, I commend the authors for their meticulous research and dedication to this field. This book is a testament to the transformative power of technology in healthcare and serves as a guidepost for those committed to advancing patient's care through innovation. I encourage every physician, researcher, and healthcare professional to engage with this text as we move forward in an era defined by the intelligent application of AI in medicine.

Peter Schwarz
MD MBA PhD
Head of the Division for Prevention and Care of Diabetes
President of the International Diabetes Federation (IDF)

Foreword

The intersection of artificial intelligence (AI) and healthcare marks a defining chapter in modern medicine, a shift that holds the potential to fundamentally transform clinical practice and patient's care. It is with great enthusiasm that I write the foreword to *Decoding Artificial Intelligence for Physicians*, a work that represents a thorough exploration of AI's role in medicine and its implications for future practice. As President of the Indian Academy of Diabetes, President of the Indian Thyroid Society, and having had the privilege to serve as the Past President of the Research Society for the Study of Diabetes in India (RSSDI) and the Association of Physicians of India (API), I have long advocated for the integration of technology to improve clinical outcomes and patient's well-being.

This book, authored by Dr Shambo Samrat Samajdar, Dr Amit Kumar Dey, and Dr Bharat Saboo, arrives at a pivotal moment when the world of healthcare is navigating complex challenges. The authors have crafted a comprehensive guide that not only explains the foundations of AI and its multifaceted applications but also addresses the practicalities of implementation and the ethical questions it raises. The content is meticulously designed to bridge the gap between theoretical AI concepts and practical, real-world applications, making it a valuable resource for physicians, researchers, and medical students.

In the realm of diabetes and metabolic disorders, which I am particularly passionate about, AI has proven to be an invaluable tool. From early detection and risk assessment to personalized management plans and patient's adherence strategies, AI offers opportunities to revolutionize how we manage chronic diseases that demand constant attention and multifactorial interventions. This book delves into how AI is transforming specialties like endocrinology, among many others, providing insights that extend beyond traditional care models. It equips physicians with the knowledge needed to incorporate AI in a way that complements human expertise, enhances diagnostic accuracy, and ultimately improves patient outcomes.

Artificial intelligence's promise does not come without challenges. Issues of data security, algorithmic bias, and the need for clear regulatory frameworks must be acknowledged and addressed to harness AI responsibly and effectively. What makes *Decoding Artificial Intelligence for Physicians* particularly noteworthy is that it does not shy away from these discussions. The authors emphasize the importance of ethical considerations, the need for clinician oversight, and the value of transparent collaboration between medical professionals and technology developers. This balanced approach ensures that readers are not only prepared to use AI but are equipped to do so in a manner that respects patient's autonomy and adheres to the highest standards of medical practice.

The inclusion of case studies and practical examples adds immense value, as these scenarios provide real-world context to the theoretical knowledge presented. Additionally, the final chapter's multiple-choice questions are an excellent tool for postgraduate students and professionals who wish to test their understanding and readiness to integrate AI into their clinical practice.

I have seen firsthand how technology can be leveraged to address the unique challenges faced by physicians, especially in a country as diverse as India, where healthcare delivery must adapt to varied settings and patient's demographics. AI has the potential to assist clinicians in overcoming disparities in healthcare access, optimizing treatment plans, and enhancing preventive care measures. This book serves as an essential guide to understanding these applications and prepares healthcare providers to take informed steps toward adopting AI as part of their practice.

As we move toward a future where AI is an integral part of healthcare, it is imperative for medical professionals to be well-versed in both its capabilities and limitations. *Decoding Artificial Intelligence for Physicians* provides the necessary foundation and inspiration for physicians to engage with AI thoughtfully and effectively. I commend the authors for their dedication to creating a resource that will undoubtedly be a guiding light for those who wish to integrate cutting-edge technology into their clinical practice for the betterment of patient's care.

Shashank R Joshi

MD DM FICP FACP (USA) FACE (USA) FRCP (Lon, Edin, Glasg)

(Padma Shri Awardee)

President, Indian Academy of Diabetes

President, Indian Thyroid Society

Past President, Research Society for the Study of Diabetes in India (RSSDI)

Past President, Association of Physicians of India (API)

Past Dean, Indian College of Physicians

Foreword

The integration of artificial intelligence (AI) into healthcare is not just a vision of the future; it is our present reality, reshaping the ways in which we diagnose, treat, and care for patients across the globe. As Chair Elect of the International Diabetes Federation (IDF) South-East Asia Region and Secretary of Diabetes India, I have had the privilege of witnessing firsthand the profound impact that digital tools and AI have on diabetes management and broader healthcare. It is with this perspective that I am honored to write the foreword for *Decoding Artificial Intelligence for Physicians*, a book that provides an in-depth and practical guide to understanding and leveraging AI in clinical practice.

Written by Dr Shambo Samrat Samajdar, Dr Amit Kumar Dey, and Dr Bharat Saboo, this book brings together the combined expertise of these distinguished professionals to deliver a comprehensive exploration of AI's potential in medicine. Their work takes an interdisciplinary approach, covering the fundamental concepts of AI, such as machine learning and natural language processing, and moving into the applications in specialized fields such as endocrinology, cardiology, oncology, and more. This format makes the book accessible to clinicians from all backgrounds, whether they are just beginning their journey with AI or are already integrating these tools into their practice.

For diabetes care, the potential of AI cannot be overstated. Managing diabetes, a disease that affects millions worldwide and poses complex challenges, requires a multi-faceted approach. AI enables predictive analytics that can identify at-risk populations earlier, personalize treatment plans, optimize medication dosing, and monitor patients in real-time. These advances have revolutionized not only how we treat diabetes but also how we engage patients in managing their own health. This book provides valuable insights into these applications and shares real-world case studies that illustrate how AI can improve outcomes for patients with diabetes and other chronic conditions.

Yet, as AI rapidly advances, it also presents challenges that must be navigated carefully. Concerns such as data privacy, algorithmic bias, and maintaining transparency in AI decision-making processes are critical issues that physicians must understand. What sets *Decoding Artificial Intelligence for Physicians* apart is that it addresses these challenges head-on. The authors emphasize the importance of ethical considerations, collaboration between developers and medical practitioners, and maintaining a balance between technological assistance and clinical expertise. This holistic approach ensures that readers are not only equipped with knowledge but are also guided on how to implement AI in a way that is safe, effective, and patient-centered.

The book's practical approach, enriched by case studies and chapter-end assessments, makes it an excellent tool for postgraduate students, researchers, and practicing physicians. These scenarios demonstrate the real-world impact of AI across different medical disciplines and provide a balanced perspective on the benefits and limitations of AI tools. For those in leadership roles, like myself, the book offers insight into how AI can be scaled to improve healthcare delivery on a regional and global scale.

As the Past President of the Research Society for the Study of Diabetes in India (RSSDI), I have been part of numerous initiatives that have aimed to bridge the gap between innovative technology and clinical practice. This book embodies that same mission, providing a roadmap for clinicians to not only understand but effectively apply AI in their daily work. It empowers healthcare professionals to be part of this technological evolution, ensuring they are prepared to harness AI's potential for the benefit of their patients.

In closing, I congratulate Dr Shambo Samrat Samajdar, Dr Amit Kumar Dey, and Dr Bharat Saboo on their meticulous and forward-thinking contribution to the medical literature. Their dedication to creating a comprehensive and accessible resource will no doubt play an essential role in helping physicians integrate AI into practice, paving the way for more informed, precise, and compassionate patient's care.

Banshi Saboo
MD PhD
Chair Elect, International Diabetes Federation (IDF) South-East Asia Region
Secretary, Diabetes India
Past President, Research Society for the Study of Diabetes in India (RSSDI)

Foreword

The world of healthcare is on the brink of a technological transformation, with artificial intelligence (AI) playing a key role in shaping the future of clinical practice. It is with great honor and anticipation that I write this foreword for *Decoding Artificial Intelligence for Physicians*, a book that skillfully navigates the complexities of AI integration in medicine. As the Governor of the American College of Physicians (India Chapter) and President-Elect of the Research Society for the Study of Diabetes in India (RSSDI), I have witnessed how AI and advanced digital tools are poised to elevate the standards of patient's care across specialties.

The authors—Dr Shambo Samrat Samajdar, Dr Amit Kumar Dey, and Dr Bharat Saboo—have produced a comprehensive and accessible guide that not only introduces the core principles of AI but also delves into its practical applications in medical practice. This book is timely, arriving when healthcare professionals around the world are seeking innovative solutions to manage an increasing patient's load while maintaining high-quality care. From diagnostics to personalized medicine and beyond, AI has proven to be a powerful ally, empowering physicians with data-driven insights that improve patient's outcomes.

In the field of diabetes and chronic disease management, which remains a significant challenge globally and in India, AI has opened new avenues for early diagnosis, personalized treatment, and continuous patient's monitoring. The predictive power of AI helps to identify individuals at risk before they develop complications, allowing for timely interventions that were once thought impossible. This book brings these concepts to life through detailed case studies, showing how AI is already being used to tackle complex medical issues. It bridges the gap between abstract technological discussions and real-world clinical applications, making it an essential read for both beginners and seasoned practitioners.

However, as with any powerful tool, the deployment of AI in healthcare comes with its share of challenges and ethical considerations. Ensuring patient's privacy, maintaining data security, and preventing algorithmic biases are areas that require careful attention. The authors of this book do not shy away from these concerns; rather, they provide a balanced perspective that includes regulatory frameworks and ethical discussions. This comprehensive approach helps to prepare physicians not only to use AI but to do so in a manner that respects patient's dignity and upholds medical integrity.

One of the standout features of *Decoding Artificial Intelligence for Physicians* is its emphasis on collaboration. The authors stress the importance of partnerships between AI developers and healthcare professionals to create tools that are both technically sound and clinically relevant. The final chapters, which include case studies and challenging multiple-choice questions, offer a unique opportunity for readers to test their understanding and deepen their knowledge. These assessments make the book an ideal resource for postgraduate students, researchers, and healthcare providers who are eager to integrate AI into their practice.

As the President-Elect of RSSDI, I am keenly aware of the potential for AI to revolutionize diabetes care, from enhancing patient's engagement through digital tools to refining treatment plans based on predictive analytics. This book aligns perfectly with the vision of combining evidence-based medicine with cutting-edge technology to achieve better outcomes for patients.

I commend Dr Shambo Samrat Samajdar, Dr Amit Kumar Dey, and Dr Bharat Saboo for their meticulous research and dedication in compiling this invaluable resource. Their work will undoubtedly inspire physicians to explore and implement AI solutions that make clinical practice more efficient, precise, and patient-focused. As we move forward in an era defined by digital health and medical innovation, this book will serve as a guiding light for those committed to embracing the future with both confidence and caution.

Anuj Maheswari

MBBS MD (General Medicine) FACE FACP FRCP (Edin)
Fellow of American College of Endocrinology, Diabetology and Metabolic Physicians

Governor, American College of Physicians (India Chapter)
President-Elect, Research Society for the Study of Diabetes in India (RSSDI)

Preface

The healthcare landscape is rapidly transforming as artificial intelligence (AI) makes significant inroads into clinical practice, medical research, and patient's care. This book, *Decoding Artificial Intelligence for Physicians*, is crafted to serve as a comprehensive resource for healthcare professionals, researchers, and postgraduate students who aspire to understand and harness the transformative potential of AI in their clinical and research endeavors. Our aim is to bridge the gap between advanced AI technologies and practical medical applications, making complex concepts accessible to those without an extensive technical background, while offering in-depth insights for advanced practitioners.

The integration of AI in healthcare is not just a trend; it represents a fundamental shift that redefines how we diagnose, treat, and prevent diseases. From enhancing diagnostic accuracy in radiology to facilitating personalized medicine in oncology and improving chronic disease management through predictive analytics, AI is already playing a critical role in patient's care. Yet, for many physicians, understanding the nuances of AI applications, ethical implications, and integration challenges remains an obstacle. This book seeks to demystify AI for clinicians by providing a structured exploration of AI's current and potential applications across multiple specialties, supplemented with practical case studies, ethical considerations, and regulatory insights.

We have organized *Decoding Artificial Intelligence for Physicians* into chapters that sequentially build on one another, beginning with fundamental concepts in AI, machine learning, and natural language processing, and moving toward specialized applications in fields such as cardiology, neurology, oncology, and more. The text addresses both the technical and practical aspects of AI, providing readers with the knowledge needed to evaluate, implement, and benefit from AI tools in clinical settings.

Each chapter has been enriched with real-world examples, tables, and case scenarios that illustrate the impact of AI in diverse medical contexts. These scenarios are intended not only to inform but also to provoke thought about the ethical, legal, and operational challenges associated with AI in healthcare. Additionally, we have included a rigorous set of multiple-choice questions in the final chapter, which serves as both a review and an advanced assessment tool, particularly for postgraduate students and medical professionals preparing for specialized examinations.

We, the authors—Dr Shambo Samrat Samajdar, Dr Amit Kumar Dey, and Dr Bharat Saboo—bring together diverse backgrounds in clinical medicine, medical research, and technological innovation. Our combined experiences across various specialties have allowed us to address AI's multidisciplinary impact on healthcare with depth and clarity. This book represents our shared commitment to equipping healthcare professionals with the tools they need to navigate the future of medicine and ultimately improve patient's outcomes through the responsible and informed use of AI.

We hope that this book will serve as a valuable guide and reference, inspiring clinicians and researchers to explore the potential of AI with a balanced perspective of its possibilities and limitations. May it empower you to embrace the future of intelligent healthcare with confidence, curiosity, and caution.

Shambo Samrat Samajdar
Amit Kumar Dey
Bharat Saboo

Contents

Introduction to Artificial Intelligence in Healthcare

INTRODUCTION

Artificial intelligence (AI) is redefining the boundaries of healthcare, transforming it from a reactive, symptom-driven discipline into a proactive, data-driven science. At its core, AI leverages algorithms and computational systems to mimic human intelligence, enabling machines to analyze vast datasets, recognize complex patterns, and make predictions that inform decision-making. Its integration into healthcare has brought a paradigm shift, promising not only enhanced diagnostic precision but also personalized care, operational efficiency, and real-time patient monitoring.

This chapter explores the foundational concepts of AI, its components, and its evolving role in modern medicine. By examining real-world applications, we aim to provide an in-depth understanding of how AI has become a cornerstone of healthcare innovation. From leveraging machine learning for predictive analytics to employing natural language processing to decipher clinical notes, AI empowers clinicians with tools that enhance their expertise, improve patient outcomes, and address systemic inefficiencies in care delivery.

The adoption of AI, however, is not without its challenges. Ethical considerations, data security, and the necessity for human oversight remain critical. This chapter also reflects on the historical evolution of AI in medicine—from early rule-based systems to today's neural networks and predictive models—highlighting its transformative potential for the future of clinical practice. By bridging the gap between advanced technologies and practical healthcare applications, AI stands as a pivotal force in redefining the way we approach medicine.

As we delve into the foundational elements of AI in healthcare, the following sections will outline its definition, key components, current applications, and the profound impact it continues to have across medical disciplines. The transformative journey of AI in healthcare is only beginning, and this chapter sets the stage for understanding its immense possibilities in shaping the future of patient care.

OVERVIEW OF ARTIFICIAL INTELLIGENCE AND ITS ROLE IN MODERN MEDICINE

Artificial intelligence (AI) has rapidly become a cornerstone technology in various sectors, with its impact profoundly felt in healthcare. AI involves creating algorithms and systems that can mimic human intelligence, learning from large volumes of data, identifying patterns, and making decisions to perform tasks that typically require human expertise. The adoption of AI in medicine has introduced transformative potential across diagnostics, treatment planning, patient monitoring, and administrative tasks, promising enhanced efficiency, accuracy, and a more personalized approach to patient care.

- *Defining AI in healthcare:* Artificial intelligence in healthcare is not a single technology but rather a suite of tools, including machine learning (ML), natural language processing (NLP), and deep learning (DL). Each of these components serves different purposes, from interpreting complex datasets to predicting disease outcomes. AI has applications in a range of healthcare activities:
  - *Diagnostics:* Leveraging imaging data for conditions, such as cancer and cardiac disease.
  - *Treatment planning:* Personalized medicine, where AI helps select treatments tailored to individual genetic profiles.
  - *Patient monitoring:* AI-driven wearable technology tracks vitals and alerts providers to critical health changes.
  - *Administrative support:* Streamlining processes, such as scheduling and billing, reducing administrative burdens.
- *Key components of AI in healthcare:*
  - *Machine learning:* ML enables computers to learn from data without explicit programming. In healthcare, ML is used to analyze patient data, predict outcomes, and identify high-risk patients. For example, ML models can predict which patients are at risk of readmission after surgery, allowing for timely interventions.
  - *Deep learning:* A subfield of ML, DL uses neural networks to process large volumes of data, particularly useful in interpreting medical images [e.g., magnetic resonance imaging (MRI) and computed tomography (CT) scans] to detect diseases.
  - *Natural language processing:* NLP is used to analyze unstructured data such as clinical notes, helping extract critical information from electronic health records (EHRs).
- *Current impact of AI in medicine:* Artificial intelligence has already demonstrated its value in healthcare settings worldwide. For instance, AI-powered diagnostic systems now assist radiologists by analyzing complex imaging data with remarkable accuracy. International Business Machines (IBM's) Watson for Oncology provides treatment recommendations based on extensive medical literature, helping oncologists develop personalized treatment plans. Additionally, in COVID-19 management, AI played a pivotal role in monitoring disease progression, tracking mutations, and even accelerating vaccine development.

EVOLUTION AND TRANSFORMATIVE POTENTIAL OF ARTIFICIAL INTELLIGENCE IN CLINICAL SETTINGS

Artificial intelligence's journey in medicine spans several decades, evolving from simple rule-based systems to complex neural networks capable of diagnosing and predicting disease outcomes with high accuracy. The transformative potential of AI in healthcare is tied to its continued evolution in the following key phases:

- *Rule-based systems (1960s–1980s):* Early AI systems relied on rule-based algorithms where computers followed a set of defined rules to solve problems. For example, MYCIN, developed in the 1970s, was an early AI system for diagnosing bacterial infections and recommending antibiotics based on clinical rules. However, rule-based systems were limited by their rigidity and inability to handle complex or novel situations, which restricted their application in medicine.

- *Emergence of ML and neural networks (1980s–2000s):* The introduction of ML algorithms enabled computers to learn from data, a major advancement from rule-based systems. Neural networks, inspired by the human brain's structure, allowed computers to identify patterns in large datasets. This era saw the development of systems, such as IBM's Deep Blue, which defeated the world chess champion in 1997, highlighting AI's potential to process information at an unprecedented scale.
- *Modern AI era (2010s–Present):* With advancements in computing power and data availability, AI has become an indispensable part of modern medicine. DL models, capable of processing vast amounts of data, revolutionized fields, such as radiology and pathology. For example, convolutional neural networks (CNNs) have been used to classify images, aiding in the detection of diseases, such as melanoma and diabetic retinopathy. AI's ability to work with large datasets also paved the way for predictive analytics in healthcare, helping clinicians anticipate complications and optimize patient outcomes.

TRANSFORMATIVE POTENTIAL OF ARTIFICIAL INTELLIGENCE IN CLINICAL PRACTICE

The potential of AI to transform healthcare lies in its ability to manage and interpret vast amounts of data, supporting clinicians with real-time insights and enabling a new era of personalized medicine. Here are key areas where AI is driving transformation in clinical settings:

- *Enhanced diagnostic accuracy:*
  - *Case scenario:* A hospital uses AI-assisted imaging to support radiologists in detecting early-stage cancers. The AI system analyzes thousands of previous cancer cases and current patient images, highlighting suspicious areas for the radiologist. This not only speeds up diagnosis but also improves accuracy, helping detect cancers at an earlier, more treatable stage.
  - *Impact:* AI-powered diagnostics can reduce diagnostic errors, often caused by human oversight, and enhance early detection, which is critical in diseases, such as cancer, where early intervention improves survival rates.
- *Predictive analytics for preventive care:*
  - *Case scenario:* An AI model analyzes EHR data to identify patients at high risk of developing chronic conditions, such as diabetes or heart disease. Physicians receive alerts for patients requiring lifestyle interventions or preventive measures, reducing the likelihood of disease progression.
  - *Impact:* Predictive analytics enables a shift from reactive to proactive healthcare, allowing clinicians to intervene before a condition becomes critical. This approach is particularly impactful in managing chronic diseases, where early intervention can drastically improve quality of life and reduce healthcare costs.
- *Personalized treatment plans:*
  - *Case scenario:* A cancer treatment center implements AI to match patients with the most effective therapies based on their genetic profiles and treatment histories. AI models help oncologists predict how individual patients will respond to specific treatments, enabling more targeted care.

- o   *Impact:* Personalized medicine, supported by AI, has the potential to improve treatment efficacy, reduce adverse effects, and promote better outcomes, particularly in complex conditions, such as cancer, where treatment response can vary widely among patients.
- *Operational efficiency and resource optimization:*
  - o   *Case scenario:* A busy emergency department (ED) employs an AI-driven triage system to classify incoming patients based on the urgency of their condition. The system uses patient data and historical records to prioritize high-risk cases, improving patient flow and reducing wait times.
  - o   *Impact:* AI-driven resource optimization in hospitals can lead to more efficient allocation of staff, reduced patient wait times, and improved patient satisfaction. Automating routine tasks also allows healthcare providers to focus on direct patient care, addressing the physician burnout crisis.
- *Artificial intelligence in remote and continuous monitoring:*
  - o   *Case scenario:* AI-enabled wearable devices continuously monitor a patient's vital signs and physical activity. If signs of a possible cardiac event are detected, the device alerts the patient and healthcare provider, prompting immediate action.
  - o   *Impact:* Continuous monitoring with AI not only empowers patients to take control of their health but also allows for early intervention in case of abnormalities. This technology is crucial for managing chronic diseases and enabling care in remote or underserved areas.

TABLES AND DATA IN ARTIFICIAL INTELLIGENCE-DRIVEN HEALTHCARE TRANSFORMATION

Application	AI technology used	Example	Impact
Diagnostic imaging	Deep learning (CNNs)	Melanoma detection from skin images	Improved accuracy, early detection
Predictive analytics	Machine learning models	Predicting hospital readmission risk	Proactive patient care, reduced costs
Personalized medicine	Genetic analysis, ML	Selecting cancer treatment based on genetic profile	Targeted therapy, better outcomes
Resource optimization	NLP, predictive analytics	Automating patient triage in emergency departments	Enhanced operational efficiency
Remote monitoring	Wearable AI, Internet of Things (IoT)	Monitoring chronic disease patients via wearables	Continuous care, reduced hospital visits

FUTURE DIRECTIONS

As AI continues to evolve, its applications in healthcare are expected to expand even further. Some anticipated advancements include the following:

- *Artificial intelligence in genomic medicine*: Integration of AI with genetic data could further enhance personalized medicine, providing insights into individual risk factors and ideal treatment protocols based on genetic markers.
- *Robotic surgery and augmented reality*: AI-powered robotic systems are expected to become more sophisticated, aiding surgeons with precision tasks. Additionally, augmented reality (AR) could provide real-time guidance during surgeries.

- *Digital therapeutics and virtual health assistants*: AI-powered virtual assistants will continue to evolve, offering patients instant access to healthcare guidance and mental health support, potentially easing the burden on healthcare providers.

CONCLUSION

Artificial intelligence is poised to revolutionize healthcare, bringing benefits that extend beyond diagnostics and treatment to reshaping healthcare delivery models. The role of AI in modern medicine continues to grow as new algorithms are developed and tested. However, it is essential to implement AI in a way that complements human expertise, with careful consideration for ethical, legal, and data privacy issues. Physicians and healthcare providers who embrace AI's transformative potential can leverage this technology to deliver high-quality, patient-centered care.

2 Fundamentals of Artificial Intelligence: Machine Learning, Deep Learning, and Natural Language Processing

INTRODUCTION

Artificial intelligence (AI) in healthcare comprises several key technologies that facilitate data-driven decision-making and clinical support for physicians. Among the most impactful components of AI are machine learning (ML), deep learning (DL), and natural language processing (NLP). Each technology has unique capabilities, enabling applications from diagnostic imaging to electronic health record (EHR) data analysis. This chapter provides a comprehensive overview of these fundamental AI technologies, examining their underlying concepts, healthcare applications, and specific algorithms relevant to physicians.

KEY CONCEPTS AND APPLICATIONS IN HEALTHCARE

Artificial intelligence's application in healthcare relies heavily on its core technologies—ML, DL, and NLP—which together enable enhanced diagnostic accuracy, predictive analytics, personalized care, and streamlined clinical workflows.

Machine Learning: Predicting Outcomes and Supporting Decision-Making

Machine learning is an AI technique in which algorithms are trained on data to recognize patterns and make predictions or decisions without being explicitly programmed. ML models range from simple linear regressions to complex ensemble models, capable of handling large datasets, extracting insights, and making recommendations.

- *Applications of ML in healthcare:*
  - Predictive analytics: ML algorithms help predict patient outcomes, including the likelihood of readmission, risk of disease progression, and potential for treatment success.
  - Clinical decision support: ML models can recommend diagnostic pathways or treatment options based on similar cases.
  - Risk stratification: ML enables physicians to identify high-risk patients based on historical data, such as patients with a high probability of complications postsurgery.
- *Case scenario:* A healthcare system implemented an ML model to predict patient readmissions. By analyzing patient demographics, past medical history, and admission data, the model accurately identified patients at risk of readmission, prompting timely interventions.

Deep Learning: Enhancing Diagnostic Accuracy and Image Analysis

Deep learning is a subset of ML that utilizes neural networks with multiple layers (hence "deep") to analyze data, particularly unstructured data, such as images and speech. DL algorithms are ideal for tasks, such as image classification and speech recognition, which are common in medical imaging and diagnostic fields.

- *Applications of DL in healthcare:*
  - Medical imaging: DL algorithms are highly effective in analyzing radiology images [e.g., computed tomography (CT), magnetic resonance imaging (MRI), X-ray] for conditions, such as cancer, fractures, and lung diseases.
  - Pathology: DL models can identify patterns in pathology slides, assisting in cancer detection and grading.
  - Speech and voice recognition: DL-based NLP models aid in transcribing patient notes and supporting virtual consultations.
- *Case scenario:* A hospital utilized a DL algorithm to screen mammograms. The model, trained on thousands of labeled images, detected early-stage breast cancer with high accuracy, aiding radiologists in timely diagnosis and improving patient outcomes.

Natural Language Processing: Extracting Insights from Textual Data

Natural language processing, a field within AI, focuses on the interaction between computers and human language. In healthcare, NLP is particularly valuable for processing unstructured data from EHRs, clinical notes, and research publications.

- *Applications of NLP in healthcare:*
  - Electronic health record data extraction: NLP algorithms help extract clinical insights from unstructured EHR text, including patient history and medication details.
  - Patient documentation and coding: NLP supports accurate medical coding by identifying key diagnostic terms in physician notes.
  - Clinical research: NLP models can rapidly analyze research papers to identify relevant studies and support evidence-based practice.
- *Case scenario:* An NLP tool was integrated into an EHR system to analyze free-text notes, automatically identifying patients with diabetes-related complications. This allowed the healthcare team to prioritize interventions, improving care outcomes for high-risk patients.

OVERVIEW OF ARTIFICIAL INTELLIGENCE ALGORITHMS RELEVANT TO PHYSICIANS

Various AI algorithms underpin the applications discussed above. The selection of an algorithm depends on the type of data, desired outcomes, and available resources. Here, we review some of the most relevant algorithms for healthcare applications.

Supervised Learning Algorithms

Supervised learning algorithms are trained on labeled data, where each input has a corresponding output. This approach is well-suited for tasks with clear data patterns, such as disease diagnosis.

- *Linear regression:*
  - Used to predict continuous outcomes, such as patient survival rates based on various predictors.
  - Example: Predicting a patient's length of stay based on age, diagnosis, and comorbidities.
- *Logistic regression:*
  - Common in binary classification tasks, logistic regression predicts the probability of an outcome (e.g., disease or no disease).
  - Example: Predicting the likelihood of a heart attack based on patient history and health metrics.
- *Decision trees and random forests:*
  - Decision trees create a model by splitting data into branches, each representing a decision rule. Random forests improve upon this by combining multiple decision trees.
  - Example: Identifying patients at high risk for diabetes complications by analyzing health records.
- *Support vector machines (SVMs):*
  - Support vector machines s are effective in high-dimensional spaces and are often used for classification tasks.
  - Example: Classifying types of skin lesions from dermatological images.

Algorithm	Application in healthcare	Strengths
Linear regression	Predicting patient outcomes (e.g., blood pressure, cholesterol levels)	Simple, interpretable
Logistic regression	Binary classification (e.g., disease presence)	Effective for clear yes/no predictions
Decision trees	Risk stratification, treatment selection	Easily interpretable, useful for decision-making
SVM	Medical image classification	High accuracy in complex classification tasks

Unsupervised Learning Algorithms

Unsupervised learning models work with unlabeled data, identifying hidden patterns or groups within data.

- *Clustering (e.g., K-means):*
  - Clustering algorithms group similar data points together, helpful for patient segmentation.
  - Example: Identifying subtypes of patients with diabetes for tailored treatment approaches.
- *Principal component analysis (PCA):*
  - Principal component analysis reduces the dimensionality of data, making complex datasets easier to analyze.
  - Example: Simplifying genetic data for cancer risk prediction models.

Deep Learning Algorithms

Deep learning models, especially neural networks, are particularly suited to processing large, unstructured datasets, such as images or text.

- *Convolutional neural networks (CNNs):*
  - Convolutional neural networks are a type of neural network optimized for image data, with applications in radiology and dermatology.

- o Example: Detecting lung cancer in CT scans or identifying melanoma from skin images.
- *Recurrent neural networks (RNNs):*
  - o Recurrent neural networks are suited for sequential data and are used in time-series analysis.
  - o Example: Predicting disease progression over time or monitoring heart rate patterns.
- *Autoencoders:*
  - o Used for data compression and anomaly detection.
  - o Example: Detecting rare genetic markers in large genomic datasets.

Deep learning algorithm	Application in healthcare	Example
CNN	Image classification	Cancer detection in radiology
RNN	Sequential data analysis	Monitoring vitals in real-time
Autoencoder	Anomaly detection	Identifying rare biomarkers in genetic data

Natural Language Processing Techniques

In addition to specific algorithms, NLP relies on techniques that facilitate text analysis, especially valuable for extracting clinical insights from unstructured data.

- *Tokenization:* Splitting text into smaller parts (tokens) to make it analyzable.
  - o Application: Breaking down physician notes into meaningful words or phrases for analysis.
- *Named entity recognition (NER):* Identifying specific terms (e.g., diseases, symptoms) within text.
  - o Example: Extracting mentions of diabetes and related symptoms from patient notes.
- *Sentiment analysis:* Identifying the emotional tone of text, used in patient feedback and mental health applications.
  - o Example: Monitoring patient interactions for signs of depression or anxiety.

CASE SCENARIOS ILLUSTRATING ARTIFICIAL INTELLIGENCE ALGORITHMS IN ACTION

- *Predictive modeling in cardiovascular care:* A hospital uses logistic regression and decision tree models to predict patients at risk of heart attacks. By analyzing health records, including cholesterol levels, lifestyle factors, and family history, the model accurately identifies high-risk patients and suggests preventive measures. This leads to improved outcomes through timely lifestyle interventions and medical checkups.
- *Cancer detection with CNNs in radiology:* A healthcare facility adopts CNN algorithms to analyze CT scans for lung cancer. The CNN model, trained on millions of images, can identify cancerous nodules with high precision, assisting radiologists in confirming diagnoses. This technology reduces diagnostic delays and improves early detection rates.
- *Natural language processing for EHR data extraction in diabetes management:* A diabetes care center integrates an NLP model with its EHR system. The NLP tool identifies high-risk patients based on unstructured physician notes, noting mentions of symptoms, such as blurred vision or increased thirst. This insight allows care teams to proactively manage high-risk patients and prevent disease complications.

FUTURE DIRECTIONS FOR ARTIFICIAL INTELLIGENCE IN HEALTHCARE

- *Integration of self-learning algorithms for autonomous updates:* Future AI systems can incorporate self-learning capabilities to autonomously update their knowledge base by analysing new medical data without requiring complete retraining.
- *Development of specialized algorithms for rare and complex diseases:* Focus on creating niche algorithms tailored to specific rare or complex conditions that are currently underserved by existing AI models. These specialized tools can utilize transfer learning and advanced clustering techniques to maximize utility from limited data sources.
- *Advanced real-time multimodal analytics:* Establish AI systems that combine data from diverse modalities in real time, such as wearable sensor outputs, genetic profiles, and imaging data. This will enable clinicians to receive comprehensive insights into a patient's condition dynamically, supporting highly personalized interventions.

CONCLUSION

The fundamentals of AI—ML, DL, and NLP—equip healthcare providers with powerful tools for transforming patient care. Each technology has unique strengths, enabling physicians to tackle complex problems, from diagnostics to predictive analytics and patient management. By leveraging these AI technologies responsibly and effectively, healthcare professionals can significantly enhance the quality of care, reduce errors, and improve patient outcomes. However, for successful integration, it is crucial for physicians to understand the capabilities and limitations of each AI technique, ensuring that they are used as complementary tools that enhance, rather than replace, human expertise.

Artificial Intelligence in Diagnostics

INTRODUCTION

Artificial intelligence (AI) has rapidly become an essential tool in the field of diagnostics, offering innovative solutions that enhance the accuracy, speed, and efficiency of disease detection. From imaging to predictive analytics, AI applications are revolutionizing diagnostics across a wide spectrum of diseases. AI's capabilities range from processing vast datasets and identifying patterns to enhancing clinicians' ability to make faster and more accurate decisions. In this chapter, we explore how AI is applied in diagnostics, examining specific case studies and evaluating its transformative impact across several diseases.

ARTIFICIAL INTELLIGENCE FOR DISEASE DETECTION AND DIAGNOSTICS

Artificial intelligence's strength in diagnostics lies in its ability to analyze complex datasets and identify patterns that may be imperceptible to human eyes. This capacity has profound implications for early disease detection, aiding in the diagnosis of conditions, such as cancer, cardiovascular disease (CVD), neurological disorders, and infectious diseases.

Artificial Intelligence in Medical Imaging

Medical imaging has been one of the earliest and most impactful areas of AI implementation in diagnostics. AI algorithms, particularly those based on deep learning, are trained to process and interpret imaging data, such as X-rays, magnetic resonance imagings (MRIs), computed tomography (CT) scans, and ultrasound images.

- *Radiology:* AI has become an invaluable asset in radiology, assisting radiologists in detecting abnormalities in medical images more accurately and quickly. For example, AI can identify nodules in lung CT scans, aiding in the early detection of lung cancer.
- *Pathology:* Digital pathology involves using AI algorithms to analyze histopathology slides for disease diagnosis. AI's ability to detect cancerous cells and grade tumors has improved accuracy, particularly in identifying early-stage cancers.
- *Cardiology:* AI is used in interpreting echocardiograms, detecting heart conditions, and predicting cardiovascular events. AI-powered electrocardiogram (ECG) interpretation tools are also helping in diagnosing arrhythmias and other cardiac issues with high accuracy.

Artificial Intelligence in Genetic and Genomic Diagnostics

In genetics and genomics, AI facilitates the analysis of vast genetic data to identify mutations linked to various diseases. AI-driven tools are increasingly used in cancer genomics, where they help identify genetic mutations that guide personalized treatment plans.

- *Genomic sequencing:* AI aids in analyzing sequences to detect disease-causing mutations, particularly for genetic disorders and cancer. In oncology, AI is used to interpret tumor genetic profiles, helping oncologists identify actionable mutations.

Predictive Diagnostics and Early Disease Detection

Artificial intelligence excels in predictive diagnostics, where algorithms analyze patient data, including medical history and lifestyle factors, to predict the likelihood of developing specific diseases. This approach enables proactive healthcare, allowing early intervention to prevent or delay disease onset.

- *Diabetes and cardiovascular diseases:* AI models analyze a patient's lifestyle, genetic predispositions, and other health metrics to predict the risk of diseases, such as diabetes and heart disease.
- *Neurodegenerative disorders:* AI-driven models predict the likelihood of developing diseases, such as Alzheimer's by analyzing biomarkers and cognitive data.

Natural Language Processing in Diagnostics

Natural Language Processing (NLP) helps extract critical information from unstructured data sources, such as physician notes, research articles, and electronic health records (EHRs). NLP tools support diagnostic processes by automatically identifying symptoms, medical histories, and risk factors in patient records, enabling quicker diagnosis.

- *Case scenario:* A hospital implemented an NLP tool to scan EHR notes for symptoms of sepsis. The tool flagged high-risk patients in real time, alerting clinicians to initiate immediate treatment, reducing sepsis mortality rates.

CASE STUDIES: ACCURACY IMPROVEMENTS IN DIAGNOSTICS ACROSS VARIOUS DISEASES

The application of AI in diagnostics has led to substantial improvements in accuracy across a range of diseases. Here, we discuss several case studies highlighting how AI enhances diagnostic precision, leading to better patient outcomes.

Artificial Intelligence in Breast Cancer Detection

- *Background:* Breast cancer is one of the most common cancers among women worldwide. Early detection significantly improves survival rates, but mammogram interpretation can be challenging, with high false positive and negative rates.
- *Artificial intelligence application:* AI algorithms have been developed to analyze mammogram images, identifying potential malignancies with greater accuracy. These algorithms, often based on convolutional neural networks (CNNs), are trained on extensive datasets of labeled mammograms, learning to distinguish benign from malignant tissue.

- *Outcome:* Studies show that AI algorithms can reduce false negatives in mammography, improving early detection rates. For example, Google Health's AI model for breast cancer screening demonstrated a reduction in false positives by 5.7% and false negatives by 9.4%, making it a powerful tool for assisting radiologists in breast cancer detection.

Metric	Traditional mammography	AI-assisted mammography
False positive rate	Higher	Reduced by 5.7%
False negative rate	Higher	Reduced by 9.4%
Diagnostic accuracy	Lower	Higher

- *Case scenario:* A hospital integrated AI into its mammography screening program. Radiologists worked with AI-generated risk scores, which identified suspicious areas that might otherwise go undetected. Over six months, early cancer detection rates improved, leading to timely treatment for several patients.

Artificial Intelligence in Lung Cancer Screening

- *Background:* Lung cancer is the leading cause of cancer-related deaths globally. Early-stage lung cancer detection through CT scans can improve survival rates, but radiologists often face challenges in identifying small nodules accurately.
- *Artificial intelligence application:* AI tools for lung cancer screening use deep learning to analyze CT scans and detect small nodules. These models are trained to recognize the distinct shapes and textures associated with cancerous growths.
- *Outcome:* A study by the National Cancer Institute demonstrated that AI could detect lung nodules with accuracy comparable to experienced radiologists. In cases of ambiguous findings, AI-assisted tools can prioritize cases requiring immediate review.

Metric	Traditional CT scan review	AI-assisted CT scan review
Detection sensitivity	Lower	Higher
Early detection rate	Moderate	Significantly improved

- *Case scenario:* A radiology department adopted an AI tool to assist in lung cancer screening. Radiologists reviewed AI-flagged images with potential nodules, resulting in faster diagnosis and reduced rates of missed early-stage cancers.

Artificial Intelligence in Cardiovascular Diagnostics

- *Background:* CVDs are a leading cause of death, with timely diagnosis crucial for managing heart disease effectively. Traditional methods, such as ECG interpretation can be prone to errors, especially in detecting subtle arrhythmias.
- *Artificial intelligence application:* AI models, particularly using deep learning, can analyze ECG data with high precision. Algorithms identify abnormal heart rhythms and subtle signs of myocardial infarction (heart attack) and atrial fibrillation (AF).
- *Outcome:* A study showed that AI-based ECG interpretation tools improved arrhythmia detection by up to 30% compared to standard methods. The Mayo Clinic's AI model for detecting asymptomatic left ventricular dysfunction demonstrated a predictive accuracy rate of over 90%.

Metric	Traditional ECG interpretation	AI-assisted ECG interpretation
Arrhythmia detection rate	Lower	Improved by up to 30%
Predictive accuracy [left ventricular (LV) dysfunction]	Moderate	Over 90%

- *Case scenario:* A cardiology unit incorporated an AI-powered ECG interpretation tool to aid in arrhythmia detection. Over 6 months, physicians identified a significant number of previously undiagnosed AF cases, enabling earlier intervention.

Artificial Intelligence in Ophthalmology: Diabetic Retinopathy Detection

- *Background:* Diabetic retinopathy is a complication of diabetes that can lead to blindness if not detected early. Screening typically involves retinal imaging, which can be time-consuming and subject to variability in interpretation.
- *Artificial intelligence application:* AI-based retinal image analysis, such as Google's DeepMind's retinal scan algorithms, detects signs of diabetic retinopathy with high sensitivity and specificity. Trained on thousands of images, these models can accurately grade the severity of retinopathy.
- *Outcome:* AI has demonstrated remarkable accuracy in detecting diabetic retinopathy, with some models achieving a sensitivity rate above 90%. AI systems can assist ophthalmologists in large-scale screening programs, helping to prevent vision loss in diabetic patients.

Metric	Traditional retinal screening	AI-assisted screening
Sensitivity for diabetic retinopathy (DR) detection	Moderate	Above 90%
Screening time	Longer	Reduced

- *Case scenario:* A diabetic clinic implemented an AI tool for screening diabetic retinopathy. Patients were scanned, and the AI flagged those requiring immediate follow-up. The clinic saw a reduction in severe retinopathy cases, as patients received timely intervention.

Artificial Intelligence in Infectious Disease Diagnostics

- *Background:* Rapid diagnosis is crucial for managing infectious diseases and preventing outbreaks. Traditional methods, such as laboratory cultures, can be slow and are often dependent on the availability of skilled personnel.
- *Artificial intelligence application:* AI models that analyze genomic sequencing data can identify pathogens quickly, helping in diagnosing infections, such as tuberculosis, human immunodeficiency virus (HIV), and COVID-19. Additionally, AI-driven chest X-ray interpretation for COVID-19 detection demonstrated promise in early screening.
- *Outcome:* AI applications in infectious disease diagnostics have led to faster turnaround times and more accurate detection of pathogens, even in low-resource settings. AI models for COVID-19 diagnosis, for example, achieved an accuracy rate of 96% in identifying positive cases based on chest imaging.

Metric	Traditional diagnostic methods	AI-assisted diagnostics
Turnaround time	Longer	Significantly reduced
Diagnostic accuracy	Moderate	Up to 96%

- *Case scenario:* During the COVID-19 pandemic, a hospital used an AI model to analyze chest X-rays for COVID-19 diagnosis. With AI assistance, clinicians could quickly triage suspected cases, speeding up diagnosis and reducing testing backlogs.

Future Directions in Healthcare

- *Real-time AI for rapid disease detection:* Develop AI models capable of analyzing diagnostic data in real-time to identify critical conditions, reducing the time to treatment in emergency scenarios.
- *Integrated diagnostic platforms:* Combine imaging, genomic, and clinical data into unified diagnostic platforms for holistic patient assessments.
- *AI-enhanced home diagnostic kits:* Expand the use of AI in home-based diagnostic kits to enable early disease detection in underserved populations.

CONCLUSION

Artificial intelligence has revolutionized diagnostics by offering tools that increase accuracy, reduce time, and enhance the ability to detect diseases early. Across diverse applications, from radiology and pathology to genetics and infectious diseases, AI supports healthcare providers by automating complex tasks and offering predictive insights that improve patient outcomes. As AI technology continues to advance, it is expected that diagnostic tools will become even more accurate, accessible, and integral to clinical practice.

4

Personalized Medicine and Clinical Decision Support with Artificial Intelligence

INTRODUCTION

Personalized medicine is an innovative approach to health care that tailors treatment plans based on individual characteristics, including genetic, environmental, and lifestyle factors. In recent years, artificial intelligence (AI) has played a significant role in advancing personalized medicine, moving away from a "one-size-fits-all" approach to a more targeted strategy for diagnosis and treatment. This chapter explores how AI is transforming precision medicine and clinical decision support (CDS), enabling healthcare providers to make more informed, timely, and individualized treatment decisions.

ARTIFICIAL INTELLIGENCE'S ROLE IN PRECISION MEDICINE AND INDIVIDUALIZED TREATMENT

Artificial intelligence's integration into personalized medicine has revolutionized how patient data is interpreted, from genetic profiles to lifestyle habits. By analyzing massive datasets, AI algorithms can identify unique patterns that inform a patient's predisposition to certain diseases, predict responses to treatment, and recommend personalized interventions.

Genomics and Precision Medicine

Genomics—the study of an individual's genetic material—provides a foundation for personalized medicine, allowing clinicians to understand the genetic basis of diseases and tailor treatments accordingly. AI excels in genomics by analyzing large-scale genetic data to identify variations and mutations that influence disease susceptibility and treatment efficacy.

Example application: In oncology, AI analyzes tumor genetic profiles to recommend targeted therapies based on specific mutations. Precision oncology has led to personalized cancer treatments that improve outcomes by targeting the molecular characteristics of each patient's cancer.

Key Techniques in Genomic Analysis

- *Deep learning for sequence analysis*: AI models process genetic sequences to identify mutations associated with diseases, such as cancer and rare genetic disorders.
- *Cluster analysis*: AI groups similar genetic profiles, helping identify subtypes within diseases, such as distinct molecular subtypes of breast cancer, each of which may respond differently to various therapies.

AI technique	Application in genomics	Impact on personalized medicine
Deep learning	Mutation detection, cancer genomics	Improved disease understanding and therapy matching
Cluster analysis	Subtype classification (e.g., in cancer)	Enables specific treatments based on cancer subtypes
Predictive modeling	Genetic predisposition analysis	Assesses patient risk and supports preventive interventions

Pharmacogenomics and Drug Response Prediction

Pharmacogenomics focuses on how genetic variations affect an individual's response to medications. AI plays a pivotal role in this field by predicting how different patients metabolize and respond to drugs, allowing for more effective, safe, and individualized drug prescriptions.

- *Example application*: AI-driven pharmacogenomic platforms analyze genetic data to predict adverse reactions or ineffective responses to medications. This application is crucial in fields, such as oncology, cardiology, and psychiatry, where incorrect drug choices or dosages can lead to severe side effects.
- *Case scenario*: A patient with a history of adverse reactions to antidepressants undergoes genetic testing. AI analyzes the patient's genotype and recommends a specific SSRI (selective serotonin reuptake inhibitor) that the patient is less likely to react negatively to, improving treatment adherence and outcomes.

Application	Impact
Predicting adverse drug reactions	Reduced side effects, improved safety
Optimizing dosage	Avoids overdosing or underdosing, enhancing efficacy
Drug selection for effectiveness	Matches patients with the most effective medications

Disease Prediction and Preventive Medicine

Artificial intelligence's predictive capabilities extend beyond treatment selection to identifying patients at risk of developing specific conditions. By analyzing genetic, lifestyle, and health data, AI models predict a patient's likelihood of developing diseases, such as diabetes, cardiovascular diseases, and neurodegenerative disorders.

- *Example application*: AI models analyze biomarkers, lifestyle data, and family history to predict diabetes risk, allowing for early intervention through lifestyle modification and preventive medication.
- *Case scenario*: A healthcare provider uses an AI-driven predictive model for diabetes. The model identifies high-risk patients based on genetic markers and lifestyle factors, enabling the clinic to offer personalized counseling on diet and exercise, potentially preventing disease onset.

Immunotherapy and Cancer Treatment

Immunotherapy, a treatment that harnesses the body's immune system to fight cancer, has shown promise in oncology. However, predicting which patients will respond to immunotherapy is challenging. AI's ability to analyze tumor genetics and the immune system has enabled more accurate predictions regarding immunotherapy response.

Example application: AI identifies biomarkers that predict patient response to immune checkpoint inhibitors, a common form of immunotherapy. This helps oncologists determine which patients are most likely to benefit, optimizing treatment plans, and reducing unnecessary side effects.

Treatment	AI role	Benefit
Immunotherapy	Predicts response to immune checkpoint inhibitors	Identifies responders, improving treatment efficacy
Chemotherapy	Determines optimal dosage, minimizing toxicity	Tailors treatment, reducing adverse effects

CLINICAL DECISION-MAKING ENHANCEMENTS THROUGH ARTIFICIAL INTELLIGENCE

Clinical decision support is a critical aspect of patient care, assisting physicians in making evidence-based decisions. AI-enhanced CDS systems bring data-driven insights to clinicians at the point of care, supporting diagnostic accuracy, treatment planning, and overall patient management.

Diagnostic Support

Artificial intelligence's role in diagnostic support involves analyzing medical imaging, laboratory results, and patient data to detect abnormalities and support differential diagnoses.
- *Imaging diagnostics*: AI-based imaging tools assist radiologists by detecting early signs of conditions, such as cancer, cardiovascular disease, and neurological disorders in magnetic resonance imaging (MRI), computed tomography (CT), and X-ray images.
- *Laboratory data interpretation*: AI algorithms analyze complex lab results, such as blood panels, to identify biomarkers indicative of diseases, such as diabetes, liver disease, or infection.
- *Case scenario*: A radiology department integrates AI tools for mammogram analysis. The AI highlights suspicious areas, supporting radiologists in identifying early-stage breast cancer, and enabling timely treatment.

Predictive Modeling in Clinical Decision Support

Predictive modeling is a cornerstone of AI-driven CDS, providing clinicians with probabilistic insights into patient outcomes. These models can predict disease progression, potential complications, and likelihood of response to treatment.
- *Example application*: In cardiology, AI-predictive models assess patient data to estimate the risk of heart failure, guiding preventive interventions.
- *Case scenario*: A cardiologist uses an AI model to predict the risk of heart failure in patients with high blood pressure. The model flags high-risk patients, prompting immediate lifestyle, and medication adjustments to mitigate the risk.

Use case	AI role	Impact
Heart failure risk assessment	Predicts patient risk based on clinical data	Enables preventive measures, improving outcomes
Diabetes progression prediction	Estimates likelihood of complications	Supports early intervention and targeted management

Real-time Decision Support in Emergency Medicine

Artificial intelligence-driven CDS systems are particularly valuable in emergency settings, where quick, data-informed decisions are critical. Real-time decision support aids in triaging, diagnostics, and treatment prioritization.

- *Example application*: In emergency rooms (ER), AI algorithms analyze vital signs and medical history to prioritize patients based on severity. These systems can alert physicians to signs of critical conditions, such as sepsis, where early intervention is crucial.
- *Case scenario*: An ER integrates an AI-based sepsis detection model. As patients enter, the model monitors vital signs and electronic health record (EHR) data, flagging those at risk of sepsis. Clinicians prioritize these patients, leading to earlier intervention and reduced mortality.

Condition	AI role	Outcome
Sepsis	Early detection and alerting	Improved survival rates through timely intervention
Cardiac arrest	Identifies high-risk patients	Reduces time-to-treatment for critical interventions

Drug Interaction and Adverse Event Prediction

Artificial intelligence enhances drug safety by predicting potential adverse drug reactions (ADRs) and interactions before they occur. This capability is especially useful for polypharmacy patients (those taking multiple medications).

- *Example application*: AI models predict drug interactions by analyzing patient medications and health conditions, alerting physicians to potential risks.
- *Case scenario*: An elderly patient is prescribed multiple medications for comorbid conditions. An AI-based CDS system reviews the medications, flagging a potential adverse interaction. The physician adjusts the treatment plan, preventing a serious drug reaction.

Use case	AI role	Impact
Polypharmacy management	Predicts adverse interactions	Enhances medication safety, reduces hospitalizations
Patient-specific dosage adjustment	Recommends safe dosages	Minimizes side effects, optimizes efficacy

Enhancing Diagnostic Accuracy through Clinical Decision Support

Artificial intelligence-powered CDS systems enhance diagnostic accuracy by analyzing symptoms, test results, and medical history to suggest potential diagnoses. These systems provide clinicians with differential diagnoses, improving diagnostic precision, especially in complex cases.

- *Example application*: In primary care, an AI CDS tool provides diagnostic suggestions based on patient symptoms and lab results. Physicians use the tool to consider rare conditions that might otherwise be overlooked.
- *Case scenario*: A primary care physician uses an AI-driven CDS system to evaluate a patient with unusual symptoms. The CDS suggests several possible diagnoses, including a rare autoimmune disorder. Further testing confirms the diagnosis, leading to early, and effective treatment.

Application	AI role	Benefit
Differential diagnosis in complex cases	Provides probable diagnoses	Reduces diagnostic errors, expedites correct diagnosis
Rare disease identification	Flags potential rare conditions	Improves outcomes through early detection

FUTURE DIRECTIONS OF ARTIFICIAL INTELLIGENCE IN PERSONALIZED MEDICINE AND CLINICAL DECISION SUPPORT

- *AI-driven polygenic risk scores:* Develop AI tools to calculate polygenic risk scores for common diseases, enabling more precise preventive measures in personalized medicine.
- *Behavorial analytics for patient engagement:* Use AI to analyze behavioral patterns and predict adherence to treatment, fostering better engagement and outcomes.
- *Dynamic drug combination optimization:* Implement AI systems to recommend optimal drug combinations based on real-time patient response data.

CONCLUSION

Artificial intelligence has significantly impacted personalized medicine and CDS, enabling healthcare providers to deliver precise, individualized care. Through applications in genomics, pharmacogenomics, predictive modeling, and real-time CDS, AI empowers clinicians with insights that enhance diagnostic accuracy, treatment efficacy, and patient safety. As AI technologies advance, their integration into clinical workflows will continue to evolve, driving a new era of personalized, data-driven health care.

In the future, AI-driven personalized medicine will likely expand further, incorporating more comprehensive datasets and offering increasingly tailored health solutions. For healthcare providers, understanding and utilizing AI-driven tools will be critical in delivering optimal, patient-centered care while maintaining ethical considerations and transparency in clinical decision-making.

Artificial Intelligence in Diabetes and Endocrinology

INTRODUCTION

Artificial intelligence (AI) is transforming diabetes and endocrinology by introducing predictive analytics, optimization tools, and personalized management strategies. In diabetes management, AI applications range from predicting disease onset to optimizing insulin dosing and monitoring. The field of endocrinology also benefits from AI in assessing and managing risks for disorders, such as thyroid disease and adrenal gland disorders. This chapter provides an in-depth exploration of AI's role in diabetes and endocrine disorder management, with a focus on predictive analytics, insulin dose optimization, and risk assessment.

PREDICTIVE ANALYTICS FOR DIABETES MANAGEMENT

Diabetes is a chronic disease that affects millions worldwide, characterized by elevated blood glucose levels. Predictive analytics in diabetes management uses AI to forecast disease progression, detect complications early, and improve overall patient outcomes.

Early Prediction of Diabetes Onset

One of AI's key roles in diabetes management is predicting the onset of type 2 diabetes (T2D) in individuals at risk. By analyzing health data, such as genetic factors, lifestyle habits, and lab results, AI models can assess an individual's risk and facilitate early intervention.

- *Example application*: AI models analyze patient history, family history, body mass index (BMI), age, and blood glucose levels to predict the likelihood of developing diabetes within a specific timeframe.
- *Case scenario*: A health clinic uses an AI-based predictive model to assess diabetes risk in patients during routine check-ups. A 45-year-old patient with a high BMI and family history of diabetes is flagged by the AI as high-risk. The clinic implements lifestyle counseling and follow-up monitoring, which helps delay the onset of diabetes.

Factors analyzed by AI	Outcome
Family history, BMI, and lifestyle	Identification of high-risk individuals
Laboratory results (HbA1c, fasting glucose)	Early diagnosis and preventive measures

Predicting Complications of Diabetes

Artificial intelligence-driven predictive models also forecast potential complications, such as cardiovascular disease, diabetic retinopathy, and kidney disease, which are common in patients with diabetes. Early prediction enables healthcare providers to tailor preventive strategies for individual patients, reducing the risk of complications.

- *Example application*: Machine learning models use data, such as HbA1c levels, cholesterol, and blood pressure to predict the likelihood of complications.
- *Case scenario*: An AI tool assesses a patient's long-term HbA1c trends, cholesterol, and blood pressure, indicating a high risk of cardiovascular complications. The healthcare provider intensifies management efforts, such as initiating medication for blood pressure and cholesterol, potentially averting future heart disease.

Complications predicted	AI-predictive factors	Preventive actions
Cardiovascular disease	HbA1c, cholesterol, and BP	Medication adjustments and lifestyle changes
Diabetic retinopathy	Duration of diabetes and blood glucose control	More frequent eye examinations
Kidney disease	Blood pressure and proteinuria	Kidney-protective interventions

Behavioral and Lifestyle Predictions

Artificial intelligence can predict patient adherence to lifestyle recommendations and medication regimes, helping providers intervene before poor compliance leads to uncontrolled blood glucose levels.

- *Example application*: AI models analyze data from wearables, such as physical activity and dietary logs, to identify patients struggling with lifestyle adherence.
- *Case scenario*: A diabetes management app utilizes AI to track patient activity and diet patterns. It notices a decline in the physical activity of a 60-year-old patient, and the AI suggests increasing engagement strategies, such as reminders and motivational messages, to help the patient adhere to exercise recommendations.

Behavior monitored	AI tool	Outcome
Physical activity	Wearable integration	Improved adherence to exercise plans
Dietary habits	Nutrition tracking	Enhanced diet compliance, better glucose control

ARTIFICIAL INTELLIGENCE IN INSULIN DOSE OPTIMIZATION AND MONITORING

Diabetes management often involves balancing insulin doses to maintain stable blood glucose levels. AI has introduced advancements in real-time insulin management through continuous glucose monitoring (CGM) systems and insulin pumps, often termed "artificial pancreas" systems.

Continuous Glucose Monitoring and Predictive Algorithms

Continuous glucose monitoring devices provide continuous blood glucose data, enabling AI algorithms to detect trends and predict future glucose levels. Predictive analytics embedded in CGMs empower patients and clinicians to anticipate blood sugar highs or lows and adjust accordingly.

- *Example application*: Machine learning models use CGM data to predict glucose levels in the next 30–60 minutes, allowing patients to adjust insulin or dietary intake proactively.
- *Case scenario*: A patient with type 1 diabetes uses a CGM device with an AI-driven app that predicts glucose trends. The app warns the patient of impending hypoglycemia, prompting them to consume carbohydrates, effectively preventing a severe hypoglycemic event.

Predictive feature	Benefit
Glucose trend analysis	Early detection of hypoglycemia/hyperglycemia
Predictive alerts	Proactive insulin or dietary adjustments

Closed-loop Insulin Delivery Systems (Artificial Pancreas)

Closed-loop insulin delivery systems use AI to analyze CGM data in real time and adjust insulin delivery through a pump without manual input. This "artificial pancreas" system mimics pancreatic function, automatically regulating blood glucose levels.

- *Example application*: AI algorithms within closed-loop systems optimize insulin dosing based on CGM data, carbohydrate intake, and physical activity, minimizing blood glucose variability.
- *Case scenario*: A patient with type 1 diabetes is equipped with an artificial pancreas that integrates CGM and insulin pump data. The AI in the system calculates insulin doses dynamically, maintaining near-normal glucose levels throughout the day with minimal manual intervention.

System feature	AI function	Outcome
Closed-loop insulin delivery	Continuous insulin adjustments	Stable glucose levels, reduced hypoglycemia risk
Personalized insulin dosing	Real-time data analysis	Improved quality of life, reduced manual dosing

Artificial Intelligence-driven Personalized Dosing Algorithms

Artificial intelligence-based personalized dosing algorithms analyze individual patient data to suggest optimal insulin doses, reducing the risks of hypoglycemia or hyperglycemia. These algorithms consider various factors, including diet, exercise, stress levels, and illness.

- *Example application*: AI-based mobile applications track patient data over time, developing personalized insulin dosing suggestions that are adaptable to lifestyle variations.
- *Case scenario*: A patient with insulin-dependent diabetes uses an AI app that integrates data on meals, exercise, and stress to calculate daily insulin requirements. The app suggests a higher dose on days when the patient's stress levels are elevated, preventing hyperglycemia.

Factors analyzed by AI	Personalized dosing outcome
Diet, exercise, and stress	Adaptive dosing, enhanced glucose control
Illness, medication interactions	Improved safety, reduced adverse events

RISK ASSESSMENT AND MANAGEMENT FOR ENDOCRINE DISORDERS

In addition to diabetes, AI aids in the diagnosis, risk assessment, and management of other endocrine disorders, including thyroid disorders, adrenal dysfunction, and hormonal imbalances.

Artificial Intelligence in Thyroid Disease Risk Assessment

Thyroid diseases, such as hypothyroidism and hyperthyroidism, are common endocrine disorders with significant health impacts. AI models use data from laboratory results, ultrasound imaging, and patient history to predict thyroid disease risk, aiding in early detection.

- *Example application*: AI algorithms analyze thyroid-stimulating hormone (TSH), T3, T4 levels, and ultrasound characteristics to classify patients at risk of thyroid disorders and suggest personalized follow-up plans.
- *Case scenario*: A clinic implements an AI tool for assessing thyroid nodules detected on ultrasound. The AI classifies nodules as benign or suspicious, helping guide the decision on whether a biopsy is necessary.

AI prediction factor	Outcome
Ultrasound characteristics	Reduces unnecessary biopsies
Laboratory values (TSH, T3, and T4)	Early diagnosis of thyroid dysfunction

Managing Adrenal Disorders with Artificial Intelligence

Adrenal disorders, including adrenal insufficiency and Cushing's syndrome, can be challenging to diagnose due to overlapping symptoms. AI helps streamline the diagnostic process by analyzing hormone levels, imaging results, and patient history.

- *Example application*: AI-driven models combine cortisol levels, adrenocorticotropin hormone (ACTH), and other endocrine tests with imaging results to predict adrenal dysfunction.
- *Case scenario*: A patient with suspected adrenal insufficiency undergoes AI-based diagnostic testing. The AI analyzes ACTH stimulation test results and cortisol levels, diagnosing the insufficiency early and allowing prompt initiation of hormone replacement therapy.

Diagnostic tool	AI role	Outcome
Cortisol and ACTH analysis	Early detection of adrenal dysfunction	Initiation of hormone therapy improved prognosis
Imaging integration	Identifies adrenal abnormalities	Enhances diagnostic accuracy

Hormonal Imbalance Risk Prediction

Artificial intelligence models assess patients for hormonal imbalances by analyzing symptoms, laboratory tests, and lifestyle factors, allowing for individualized management of endocrine-related symptoms, such as polycystic ovary syndrome (PCOS) and menopause.

- *Example application*: AI analyzes hormonal profiles, menstrual history, and metabolic markers to diagnose PCOS and predict potential complications, such as infertility or metabolic syndrome.

- *Case scenario*: An AI tool used in an endocrinology practice analyzes hormonal profiles and menstrual irregularities to diagnose PCOS. The tool also identifies high-risk patients for metabolic complications, prompting lifestyle recommendations.

Hormonal imbalance	AI assessment	Management outcome
PCOS, menopause	Risk assessment for complications	Personalized management, preventive strategies
Hormone replacement prediction	AI-guided dosing	Improved symptom control, reduced side effects

FUTURE DIRECTIONS OF ARTIFICIAL INTELLIGENCE IN DIABETES AND ENDOCRINE MANAGEMENT

- *AI in psychosocial aspects of diabetes:* Introduce AI to assess and address the emotional and psychological challenges faced by diabetes patients, improving holistic care.
- *AI-powered nutritional interventions:* Develop AI platforms to provide personalized dietary recommendations, integrating CGM data and meal logs.
- *Predictive models for diabetic complications:* Use AI to forecast the risk of specific complications (e.g., nephropathy, neuropathy) and enable preemptive interventions.

CONCLUSION

Artificial intelligence has become an indispensable tool in diabetes and endocrinology, contributing to early diagnosis, personalized management, and improved outcomes. By leveraging predictive analytics, insulin dose optimization, and risk assessment tools, AI empowers healthcare providers to deliver tailored interventions, reduce complications, and enhance patient quality of life. As AI technology advances, its application in diabetes and endocrine care will continue to expand, offering patients and providers more precise and effective solutions for managing these complex chronic conditions.

The future of AI in this field holds exciting potential, with innovations that will further refine individualized care and support clinicians in delivering optimal treatments. Ultimately, AI-driven tools and techniques will allow for a proactive, preventive, and personalized approach to diabetes and endocrine disorders, leading to better health outcomes, and more efficient care systems.

Artificial Intelligence in Cardiovascular Diseases

INTRODUCTION

Cardiovascular diseases (CVDs) remain the leading cause of death worldwide, demanding advanced tools to manage risk, diagnose conditions, and support treatment. Artificial intelligence (AI) has emerged as a powerful tool in cardiovascular medicine, providing clinicians with enhanced diagnostic accuracy, predictive capabilities, and automated support systems. In this chapter, we explore the application of AI-driven tools in cardiovascular risk assessment, arrhythmia detection, heart failure and hypertension management, and AI-assisted cardiac imaging technologies, such as echocardiography and electrocardiogram (EKG) interpretation.

ARTIFICIAL INTELLIGENCE-DRIVEN TOOLS FOR CARDIOVASCULAR RISK ASSESSMENT AND MONITORING

Predictive analytics powered by AI has become essential in identifying individuals at high risk for cardiovascular events and monitoring existing conditions. AI tools enable the analysis of large-scale datasets, including electronic health records (EHRs), genetic information, lifestyle factors, and wearable data, to assess an individual's risk profile and suggest preventive interventions.

Risk Prediction for Cardiovascular Events

Artificial intelligence algorithms analyze various data inputs to predict the risk of cardiovascular events, such as heart attacks and strokes. These models integrate diverse risk factors, such as cholesterol levels, blood pressure, age, genetic predispositions, and lifestyle factors, to provide personalized risk assessments.

- *Example application*: Machine learning algorithms use data from EHRs to evaluate a patient's likelihood of experiencing a cardiovascular event in the next 5–10 years, supporting clinicians in developing personalized prevention plans.
- *Case scenario*: A middle-aged patient undergoes a routine check-up, and an AI-driven risk assessment tool evaluates their clinical and lifestyle data. The tool identifies the patient as high risk for heart disease, prompting the physician to initiate a preventive regimen of lifestyle modifications and statin therapy.

Risk factors analyzed	AI role	Outcome
Age, cholesterol, blood pressure, and lifestyle habits	Risk prediction	Personalized preventive care
Genetic predispositions	Early detection of high-risk individuals	Improved monitoring and proactive management

Monitoring and Early Detection of Cardiovascular Disease

For patients with existing cardiovascular conditions, AI-enabled monitoring tools play a crucial role in detecting early signs of disease progression and complications. Wearable devices, combined with AI, monitor key health metrics, such as heart rate variability, blood pressure, and physical activity, providing real-time insights for both patients and clinicians.

- *Example application*: AI models analyze continuous data from wearables to detect anomalies that may indicate disease progression, allowing for timely intervention.
- *Case scenario*: A patient with hypertension wears a smart device that monitors blood pressure and heart rate. The AI system detects an upward trend in blood pressure, triggering an alert for the healthcare team. The physician adjusts the patient's medication, preventing further complications.

Metric monitored	AI role	Outcome
Blood pressure and heart rate	Trend detection and early alerting	Timely medication adjustments
Physical activity	Compliance monitoring	Improved patient adherence and engagement

APPLICATIONS IN ARRHYTHMIA DETECTION, HEART FAILURE, AND HYPERTENSION MANAGEMENT

Artificial intelligence's role in cardiovascular medicine extends to the detection and management of specific conditions, such as arrhythmias, heart failure, and hypertension. By analyzing EKG data, patient records, and health metrics, AI supports clinicians in diagnosing and managing these chronic conditions.

Arrhythmia Detection

Arrhythmias, or irregular heart rhythms, can range from benign to life-threatening. Traditional detection methods, such as Holter monitoring, are limited by their intermittent nature. AI-enhanced tools improve the detection accuracy of arrhythmias, such as atrial fibrillation (AFib), by analyzing EKG data and continuous heart rhythm monitoring.

- *Example application*: Deep-learning algorithms trained on EKG data detect AFib and other arrhythmias with higher sensitivity and specificity than traditional methods.
- *Case scenario*: A 65-year-old patient presents with occasional palpitations. Using an AI-enhanced EKG app, the clinician can analyze EKG data and detect intermittent AFib, enabling timely anticoagulation therapy to reduce stroke risk.

Arrhythmia type	AI detection tool	Outcome
Atrial fibrillation	EKG analysis	Early detection, reduced stroke risk
Ventricular arrhythmia	Continuous monitoring	Enhanced detection and prevention of cardiac events

Heart Failure Management

Heart failure is a chronic condition that requires careful monitoring and management to prevent hospitalizations and improve quality of life. AI-driven models predict the risk of heart failure in at-risk populations and monitor symptoms and biomarkers to detect early signs of decompensation.

- *Example application*: AI models analyze data from EHRs and wearable devices to detect trends indicative of heart failure exacerbations, such as weight gain, reduced physical activity, and changes in heart rate variability.
- *Case scenario*: A heart failure patient is monitored through a wearable device and an AI app that tracks weight and heart rate variability. When the AI detects early signs of fluid retention, the healthcare team increases diuretics, preventing hospital admission.

Monitoring factor	AI role	Outcome
Weight and physical activity	Early detection of fluid retention	Reduced hospitalizations
Heart rate variability	Prediction of exacerbations	Improved medication management

Hypertension Management

Hypertension, or high blood pressure, is a major risk factor for CVD and requires long-term management. AI-driven tools support blood pressure management by analyzing home monitoring data and providing tailored recommendations.

- *Example application*: AI algorithms process blood pressure readings from home-monitoring devices, suggesting lifestyle modifications, and medication adjustments as needed.
- *Case scenario*: A patient with hypertension uses a home blood pressure monitor with AI capabilities. The device detects persistently elevated readings, alerting the physician, who adjusts the patient's treatment plan to maintain target blood pressure levels.

Parameter monitored	AI tool	Outcome
Blood pressure readings	Trend analysis and medication suggestion	Optimized blood pressure control
Patient lifestyle factors	Tailored lifestyle advice	Improved long-term adherence

ARTIFICIAL INTELLIGENCE IN ECHOCARDIOGRAPHY, ELECTROCARDIOGRAM INTERPRETATION, AND OTHER CARDIAC IMAGING

Cardiac imaging is central to diagnosing and managing cardiovascular conditions. AI has significantly enhanced the interpretation of echocardiograms, EKGs, and other imaging modalities, allowing for faster and more accurate diagnoses.

Artificial Intelligence in Echocardiography

Echocardiography is a widely used imaging tool for assessing cardiac function, structure, and hemodynamics. AI models automate the interpretation of echocardiograms, assisting in identifying conditions, such as left ventricular hypertrophy, valvular disease, and reduced ejection fraction.

- *Example application*: Convolutional neural networks (CNNs) analyze echocardiographic images to quantify cardiac function and detect abnormalities with high accuracy.

- *Case scenario*: An echocardiography laboratory integrates an AI tool for automated ejection fraction measurement. The AI system flags abnormalities in a patient's heart function, enabling a cardiologist to diagnose early-stage heart failure and initiate treatment.

Echocardiographic measure	AI role	Outcome
Ejection fraction	Automated measurement	Faster, accurate diagnosis of heart failure
Valvular abnormalities	Detection and classification	Early treatment planning

Electrocardiogram Interpretation

Electrocardiograms provide valuable information on heart rhythm, electrical activity, and ischemic changes. AI-enhanced EKG interpretation improves the detection of arrhythmias, ischemia, and other conditions.

- *Example application*: AI algorithms interpret EKG data, identifying abnormalities, such as prolonged QT intervals or signs of myocardial infarction with greater accuracy and speed than traditional methods.
- *Case scenario*: An emergency department adopts an AI-based EKG interpretation tool. The system quickly flags EKGs indicative of acute myocardial infarction, enabling rapid initiation of treatment, and reducing time to intervention.

EKG parameter	AI interpretation	Outcome
QT interval	Detection of prolonged intervals	Prevention of torsades de pointes
ST-segment elevation	Rapid identification of myocardial infarction	Reduced door-to-balloon time

Artificial Intelligence in Cardiac Magnetic Resonance Imaging and Computed Tomography Imaging

Magnetic resonance imaging (MRI) and computed tomography (CT) are advanced imaging modalities for detailed assessment of cardiac structure and function. AI tools streamline image interpretation, supporting more accurate diagnoses, and reducing clinician workload.

- *Example application*: AI-driven cardiac MRI analysis enables automated segmentation of cardiac structures, facilitating accurate volume, and functional assessments.
- *Case scenario*: A patient with suspected myocarditis undergoes a cardiac MRI. An AI tool segments the myocardium and detects areas of inflammation, assisting the radiologist in diagnosing myocarditis, and guiding treatment.

Imaging modality	AI application	Outcome
Cardiac MRI	Myocardial segmentation	Accurate diagnosis of myocarditis
Cardiac CT	Coronary artery analysis	Early detection of coronary artery disease

FUTURE DIRECTIONS FOR ARTIFICIAL INTELLIGENCE IN CARDIOVASCULAR MEDICINE

- *AI in cardiovascular rehabilitation:* Integrate AI into post-event rehabilitation programs to personalize exercise regimens and monitor patient progress remotely.

- *Next-gen cardiac wearables:* Develop AI-powered wearables that monitor advanced metrics, such as myocardial strain and coronary flow dynamics.
- *Global cardiovascular risk models:* Use AI to create universally applicable risk assessment tools that incorporate diverse population data for global health impact.

CONCLUSION

Artificial intelligence is transforming CVD management by providing predictive, diagnostic, and monitoring capabilities that are essential in both preventive and acute care. From risk assessment and monitoring to arrhythmia detection, heart failure management, and cardiac imaging, AI offers significant advancements in managing and treating cardiovascular conditions. By integrating AI-driven tools, clinicians can provide more accurate, timely, and personalized care to their patients, potentially reducing mortality and improving quality of life.

As AI continues to evolve, its applications in cardiovascular medicine will become more refined, transparent, and comprehensive. Future developments will likely see AI tools that integrate multiple sources of data, from wearables and EHRs to imaging and genetic information, offering a holistic view of cardiovascular health. The continued collaboration between AI technology and clinical expertise will be crucial in ensuring that AI serves as an effective, reliable, and ethical tool in the fight against CVD.

Artificial Intelligence in Renal Diseases

INTRODUCTION

Kidney diseases are a major public health concern, often progressing silently until they reach an advanced stage. The management of renal diseases, including chronic kidney disease (CKD) and acute kidney injury (AKI), requires early detection, timely intervention, and consistent monitoring. Artificial intelligence (AI) has become a transformative force in nephrology, introducing advanced tools for early detection, prognosis, and optimization of care pathways. This chapter explores the applications of AI in detecting kidney diseases, predictive modeling for dialysis and transplant needs, and enhancing renal function monitoring to improve patient outcomes.

ARTIFICIAL INTELLIGENCE APPLICATIONS IN EARLY DETECTION AND PROGNOSIS OF KIDNEY DISEASES

Artificial intelligence's predictive and analytical capabilities make it well suited for the early detection of kidney diseases. By analyzing diverse data from electronic health records (EHRs), genetic information, and biomarkers, AI models can identify patients at risk of CKD and AKI, allowing for earlier intervention and potentially slowing disease progression.

Early Detection of Chronic Kidney Disease

Chronic kidney disease often progresses without noticeable symptoms until it reaches an advanced stage. Artificial intelligence-powered predictive models analyze patient data to assess CKD risk and provide an early warning, enabling preventive measures and monitoring.

- *Example application*: Machine learning algorithms use factors, such as age, blood pressure, glucose levels, and medical history to identify individuals at high risk of CKD, even before symptoms appear.
- *Case scenario*: A primary care clinic employs an AI-based tool for CKD risk assessment during routine checkups. The tool flags a 50-year-old patient with elevated blood pressure and a history of diabetes as high risk, prompting the clinician to initiate regular monitoring and recommend lifestyle changes to slow disease progression.

Risk factors analyzed by AI	Outcome
Blood pressure, glucose levels, and family history	Early detection and preventive care
Age, body mass index, and lifestyle factors	Identification of high-risk individuals

Predicting Acute Kidney Injury

Acute kidney injury can develop rapidly, often as a complication of other conditions, such as sepsis, surgery, or medication use. Early detection is crucial to prevent progression to CKD or even kidney failure. AI models assess real-time data to predict AKI risk, allowing for proactive management.

- *Example application*: AI models analyze factors, such as urine output, blood creatinine levels, and fluid balance to predict AKI risk in hospitalized patients, providing early alerts to healthcare teams.
- *Case scenario:* In an intensive care unit, an AI-driven AKI prediction model monitors real-time data from patient monitors. When the system detects early signs of AKI in a postoperative patient, it alerts the intensive care unit team, who adjusts medications and fluids, preventing further kidney damage.

AKI risk factors monitored	AI role	Outcome
Urine output and creatinine levels	Early warning of AKI	Prevention of progression to severe AKI
Blood pressure and medication use	Risk prediction for at-risk patients	Proactive management to mitigate kidney injury

Artificial Intelligence in Genetic Screening for Kidney Disease

Artificial intelligence is also instrumental in analyzing genetic data to identify individuals with genetic mutations that increase the risk of kidney disease. This approach is particularly beneficial for families with a history of hereditary kidney disorders, such as polycystic kidney disease.

- *Example application*: Deep learning models process genetic sequences to identify mutations linked to kidney diseases, allowing for early intervention strategies.
- *Case scenario*: A patient with a family history of polycystic kidney disease undergoes genetic screening. An AI algorithm detects a specific mutation, leading the healthcare provider to initiate preventive monitoring and provide genetic counseling for the patient's family.

Genetic markers analyzed	Outcome
Polycystic kidney disease-related mutations	Early diagnosis and preventive care
Inherited risk factors	Identification of high-risk family members

Predictive Modeling for Dialysis and Transplant Needs

As kidney disease progresses, patients may require dialysis or kidney transplantation. Predictive modeling powered by AI can forecast the need for these treatments, allowing for better resource allocation and preparation for both patients and healthcare providers.

Predicting Dialysis Onset

Artificial intelligence-driven predictive models analyze patient data to forecast the need for dialysis, helping nephrologists plan timely interventions and prepare patients for renal replacement therapy.

- *Example application*: Machine learning models assess renal function indicators, such as glomerular filtration rate (GFR), creatinine levels, and comorbidities to predict when a patient is likely to require dialysis.

- *Case scenario*: A nephrology clinic uses an AI model to monitor CKD patients' laboratory results and symptoms. The model predicts that a patient's kidney function will decline to the dialysis threshold within 6 months, allowing the care team to start preparing the patient for dialysis and explore potential access options.

Predictive factors for dialysis	AI role	Outcome
GFR, creatinine, and comorbid conditions	Forecasting dialysis needs	Early preparation and patient education
Patient symptoms and laboratory trends	Proactive planning for renal replacement	Reduced risk of emergency dialysis start

Transplant Eligibility and Prioritization

For patients who are candidates for kidney transplantation, AI models support transplant prioritization by assessing eligibility, donor-recipient matching, and predicting post-transplant outcomes. This approach can enhance allocation efficiency and improve long-term outcomes.

- *Example application*: AI algorithms analyze factors like blood type compatibility, human leukocyte antigen (HLA) matching, and predicted graft survival to prioritize candidates on the transplant list.
- *Case scenario:* A transplant center adopts an AI-based system to improve matching between donors and recipients. The AI suggests that a particular donor kidney has high compatibility with a patient, leading to a successful transplant with a reduced risk of rejection.

Transplant matching factors	AI role	Outcome
Blood type and HLA compatibility	Prioritizing transplant candidates	Optimized matching and improved graft survival
Graft survival prediction	Post-transplant planning	Reduced rejection rates and improved outcomes

Predicting Post-transplant Outcomes

Artificial intelligence models can predict the likelihood of complications following kidney transplantation, such as rejection or infection. These predictions allow clinicians to develop personalized monitoring and intervention plans.

- *Example application*: Machine learning algorithms analyze post-transplant patient data, such as immune markers and kidney function trends, to identify patients at high risk of rejection.
- *Case scenario*: *A patient* who recently received a kidney transplant is monitored through an AI model that predicts potential rejection based on immune system activity. Early warning allows clinicians to adjust immunosuppressive therapy, minimizing the risk of rejection.

Post-transplant factors monitored	AI role	Outcome
Immune markers and kidney function trends	Predicting rejection risk	Proactive adjustments to immunosuppressive therapy
Infection indicators	Early identification of complications	Reduced morbidity and improved graft function

Optimizing Renal Function Monitoring and Care Pathways

Artificial intelligence also enhances renal disease management through optimized monitoring of renal function and improved care pathways, promoting effective disease progression control and streamlined patient management.

Continuous Monitoring of Renal Function

Artificial intelligence-powered continuous monitoring tools integrate with wearable devices and mobile health applications, tracking renal function indicators, such as blood pressure, fluid intake, and laboratory results. These tools help both patients and providers stay informed of changes in renal function.

- *Example application*: AI-enabled applications analyze blood pressure and fluid balance data, providing real-time feedback and alerts for out-of-range values, thus helping patients with CKD manage their condition more effectively.
- *Case scenario*: A patient with CKD uses a wearable device connected to an AI application that monitors blood pressure and daily fluid intake. When the patient's blood pressure exceeds the recommended range, the application sends an alert to the healthcare team, who adjusts the patient's medication.

Monitoring parameter	AI role	Outcome
Blood pressure and fluid balance	Real-time monitoring and alerts	Improved blood pressure control and reduced complications
Laboratory results	Early detection of worsening renal function	Timely treatment adjustments

Dynamic Adjustment of Treatment Plans

Artificial intelligence models facilitate adaptive treatment plans based on real-time data and evolving patient needs. This is particularly valuable for patients with CKD, whose condition can fluctuate due to various factors, such as infections, diet, and medication.

- *Example application*: AI models adjust treatment plans dynamically based on renal function, medication adherence, and symptom data, ensuring optimal care.
- *Case scenario*: An AI-driven care platform for patients with CKD monitors laboratory results and symptoms, making real-time adjustments to treatment. When a patient's GFR drops suddenly, the AI suggests reducing certain medications, preventing further kidney stress.

Treatment adjustment factor	AI role	Outcome
GFR fluctuations	Real-time treatment adaptation	Reduced medication-related kidney damage
Symptom tracking	Personalized care adjustments	Improved quality of life and optimized renal function

Care Coordination and Patient Engagement

Artificial intelligence tools support coordinated care by facilitating communication between patients, nephrologists, and other healthcare providers. AI-based patient engagement applications provide educational resources, reminders, and motivational tools to improve adherence and quality of life.

- *Example application*: AI-driven apps send reminders for medication, provide dietary advice, and connect patients with healthcare teams for questions, promoting adherence and self-management.
- *Case scenario*: A patient with CKD uses an AI app that provides reminders to take medications, offers dietary guidance, and sends alerts for upcoming appointments. By following the AI-based suggestions, the patient maintains stable kidney function and experiences fewer complications.

Patient engagement tool	AI role	Outcome
Medication reminders and dietary advice	Promote adherence and education	Improves adherence and reduces disease progression
Communication platform	Connects patients with healthcare providers	Enhanced patient engagement and support

FUTURE DIRECTIONS FOR ARTIFICIAL INTELLIGENCE IN RENAL DISEASE MANAGEMENT

- *AI-powered fluid management systems:* Develop systems that use real-time patient data to optimize fluid intake and reduce risks associated with fluid overload in CKD and AKI patients.
- *Predictive analytics for graft survival:* Utilize AI to predict graft survival post-kidney transplantation, guiding personalized immunosuppressive therapy.
- *Remote biomarker monitoring devices:* Innovate wearable technology to monitor renal-specific biomarkers (e.g., creatinine, BUN) in real-time for proactive management.

CONCLUSION

Artificial intelligence has proven instrumental in transforming the detection, monitoring, and management of renal diseases, enabling early intervention, improved patient engagement, and optimized care pathways. From predicting disease onset and dialysis needs to refining post-transplant care and enhancing renal function monitoring, AI applications in nephrology support clinicians and empower patients, ultimately improving outcomes and quality of life.

The future of AI in renal diseases promises even more personalized, data-driven care, as AI systems evolve to incorporate genetic, clinical, and lifestyle data for comprehensive, individualized treatment approaches. By embracing AI-driven tools and advancements, nephrology can continue to improve the management of CKD, AKI, and other renal conditions, ultimately reducing the global burden of kidney disease.

Artificial Intelligence in Ophthalmology

INTRODUCTION

Ophthalmology, the branch of medicine focused on eye health, has seen rapid advancements with the integration of artificial intelligence (AI). AI technologies, particularly those involving machine learning and deep learning, are transforming the detection, management, and treatment of eye diseases, such as diabetic retinopathy (DR), glaucoma, and age-related macular degeneration (AMD). This chapter explores AI applications in ophthalmic imaging, diagnosis, surgical planning, and patient monitoring, providing insights into how AI improves accuracy, enhances early detection, and facilitates personalized care in ophthalmology.

ARTIFICIAL INTELLIGENCE IN THE DETECTION AND MANAGEMENT OF DIABETIC RETINOPATHY, GLAUCOMA, AND MACULAR DEGENERATION

The early detection and management of eye diseases are critical to preventing vision loss. AI applications have proven particularly valuable in identifying and monitoring conditions, such as DR, glaucoma, and macular degeneration, which require regular screening and timely intervention.

Diabetic Retinopathy Detection and Management

Diabetic retinopathy is a leading cause of blindness among individuals with diabetes, characterized by damage to the blood vessels in the retina. Early detection through regular screening is essential to prevent severe vision loss. AI-driven systems have significantly improved the detection of DR by analyzing retinal images with high accuracy, enabling early diagnosis and intervention.

- *Example application*: Deep learning models trained on large data sets of retinal images can identify signs of DR with accuracy comparable with or better than human experts.
- *Case scenario:* An ophthalmology clinic uses an AI-based retinal screening tool for diabetic patients. The AI analyzes each retinal image, identifying patients with mild or severe DR and recommending follow-up care accordingly. By streamlining screening, the clinic ensures that high-risk patients receive timely treatment, reducing the incidence of vision loss.

Retinal changes detected	AI role in detection	Outcome
Microaneurysms, hemorrhages	Automated image analysis	Early detection and intervention
Retinal neovascularization	Identification of disease progression	Timely referral to specialists

Glaucoma Detection and Monitoring

Glaucoma, often referred to as the "silent thief of sight," is a group of eye conditions that cause optic nerve damage and progressive vision loss. Traditional screening methods rely on intraocular pressure (IOP) measurement and optic nerve imaging. AI enhances glaucoma detection by analyzing optic nerve health and visual field changes with high precision.

- *Example application:* AI models analyze optical coherence tomography (OCT) images to assess optic nerve head and retinal nerve fiber layer thickness, helping detect early signs of glaucoma.
- *Case scenario:* A patient at risk of glaucoma undergoes screening with an AI-enhanced OCT scanner. The AI detects subtle thinning of the retinal nerve fiber layer, even before the patient shows symptoms. The ophthalmologist initiates IOP-lowering therapy, delaying the progression of glaucoma.

Optic nerve indicators	AI detection role	Outcome
Nerve fiber layer thinning	Early identification of glaucoma risk	Early intervention, preservation of vision
Optic disc cupping	Monitors disease progression	Personalized treatment planning

Age-related Macular Degeneration

Age-related macular degeneration is a common cause of vision impairment in older adults, affecting the central portion of the retina (macula). AI applications assist in the detection of AMD by analyzing fundus and OCT images for signs of drusen and geographic atrophy, key indicators of the disease.

- *Example application:* Machine learning algorithms assess the presence of drusen, retinal pigment changes, and fluid accumulation in OCT scans, distinguishing between dry and wet AMD.
- *Case scenario:* An AI-powered system in a vision center analyzes fundus images of an elderly patient and detects signs of early-stage AMD. The AI model classifies the AMD type and severity, prompting regular follow-up visits and guiding potential treatment with anti-vascular endothelial growth factor (anti-VEGF) therapy for wet AMD.

AMD indicators	AI role	Outcome
Presence of drusen, geographic atrophy	Early diagnosis of AMD	Prevention of severe vision loss
Fluid accumulation	Identifies wet AMD	Timely initiation of anti-VEGF therapy

ROLE OF ARTIFICIAL INTELLIGENCE IN OPHTHALMIC IMAGING AND DIAGNOSIS

Artificial intelligence has revolutionized ophthalmic imaging by enhancing the interpretation of images from various modalities, including fundus photography, OCT, and visual field testing. AI's image analysis capabilities improve diagnostic accuracy, streamline workflows, and support clinical decision-making in ophthalmology.

Fundus Photography and Automated Image Analysis

Fundus photography captures images of the retina, enabling the detection of diseases affecting the retinal structure. AI algorithms enhance fundus image analysis by detecting subtle retinal changes, providing rapid and accurate diagnosis.

- *Example application*: AI-powered fundus imaging systems identify abnormalities, such as hemorrhages, microaneurysms, and retinal detachment, supporting diagnoses for conditions like DR and hypertensive retinopathy.
- *Case scenario*: An AI-assisted fundus imaging system in a primary care setting screens patients with diabetes for retinopathy. The AI tool identifies high-risk patients and refers them for further examination, facilitating early intervention and preventing vision loss.

Condition detected by AI	AI application	Outcome
Diabetic retinopathy, retinal detachment	Automated detection of abnormalities	Faster diagnosis and referral
Hypertensive retinopathy	Identifies early retinal vascular changes	Preventive care and blood pressure management

Optical Coherence Tomography

Optical coherence tomography is an imaging technique that provides cross-sectional views of retinal layers, widely used in diagnosing retinal diseases. AI enhances OCT image interpretation, detecting pathologies, such as macular edema, retinal detachment, and structural abnormalities.

- *Example application*: AI-based OCT systems automatically segment retinal layers, measure thickness, and detect abnormalities in macular and optic nerve regions.
- *Case scenario:* A patient with suspected macular edema undergoes an OCT scan with AI-enhanced analysis. The AI identifies fluid accumulation in the macula, enabling the ophthalmologist to confirm the diagnosis and start anti-VEGF therapy, improving the patient's vision outcome.

Pathology detected by OCT	AI role	Outcome
Macular edema, retinal detachment	Automated segmentation and fluid detection	Early diagnosis and timely treatment
Optic nerve abnormalities	Structural assessment of optic disc	Improved glaucoma management

Visual Field Testing and AI Analysis

Visual field testing assesses the functional status of a patient's vision, particularly in glaucoma and neurological conditions. AI enhances the analysis of visual field test results by detecting patterns indicative of disease progression or abnormalities.

- *Example application*: Machine learning models analyze visual field patterns to detect early signs of glaucoma, supporting the classification of glaucoma stages and progression.
- *Case scenario:* A glaucoma patient undergoes visual field testing, and the AI model identifies progressive field loss consistent with glaucoma. Based on AI's assessment, the ophthalmologist intensifies treatment, preserving the patient's remaining vision.

Visual field changes detected	AI role in analysis	Outcome
Glaucoma progression	Pattern recognition of field loss	Tailored treatment plan, delayed progression
Central scotomas in macular disease	Disease monitoring	Adjusted therapy for AMD

ENHANCEMENTS IN SURGICAL PLANNING AND PATIENT MONITORING

Artificial intelligence applications extend beyond diagnostics to surgical planning and postoperative monitoring, supporting ophthalmologists in delivering more precise, effective, and personalized care.

Surgical Planning in Ophthalmology

Artificial intelligence assists in planning for eye surgeries, such as cataract extraction, retinal surgery, and refractive surgery, by simulating surgical outcomes and guiding decision-making based on individual patient data.

- *Example application:* AI-powered tools for cataract surgery planning calculate optimal intraocular lens (IOL) power, improving visual outcomes and reducing postoperative complications.
- *Case scenario:* A patient scheduled for cataract surgery undergoes preoperative screening with an AI tool that calculates IOL power based on corneal measurements and eye length. The precise IOL selection enhances visual acuity postsurgery, improving the patient's satisfaction.

Surgery type	AI Application in Planning	Outcome
Cataract surgery	IOL power calculation and alignment	Improved refractive outcomes
Refractive surgery	Customized corneal mapping	Enhanced accuracy, reduced complications

AI in Retinal Surgery and Vitrectomy

Retinal surgeries, including vitrectomy, require meticulous planning and precision. AI models assist in identifying anatomical landmarks and potential risks, supporting surgeons in achieving better outcomes.

- *Example application:* AI systems analyze preoperative retinal images to identify structural damage, guide vitrectomy planning, and predict the likelihood of complications.
- *Case scenario:* An AI-driven retinal imaging tool assesses a patient's preoperative retinal structure before a vitrectomy. The AI helps the surgeon identify areas of traction and plan the procedure, resulting in reduced risk of retinal detachment and improved visual recovery.

Surgical procedure	AI role in planning	Outcome
Vitrectomy, retinal repair	Structural mapping and complication prediction	Increased surgical precision
Laser photocoagulation	Identifies target zones	Reduces tissue damage, effective treatment

Postoperative Monitoring and Patient Engagement

Artificial intelligence-driven monitoring systems track patient progress after eye surgeries, providing alerts for potential complications and supporting continuous care. Patient engagement platforms use AI to offer tailored advice, reminders, and resources for better postoperative recovery.

- *Example application:* AI-enabled applications monitor symptoms after cataract or LASIK (laser-assisted in situ keratomileusis) surgery, reminding patients to follow care protocols and alerting clinicians to signs of complications.
- *Case scenario:* A patient who recently had cataract surgery uses an AI application to track symptoms and medication adherence. The app sends reminders for eye drops and detects potential signs of inflammation, prompting a follow-up visit to prevent complications.

Postoperative condition	AI monitoring role	Outcome
Inflammation, infection	Symptom tracking and alerting	Early intervention, reduced complications
Patient adherence	Medication reminders and follow-up alerts	Improved recovery, reduced postoperative risks

FUTURE DIRECTIONS FOR ARTIFICIAL INTELLIGENCE IN OPHTHALMOLOGY

- *AI-powered wearable devices for continuous monitoring:* Develop smart wearable devices integrated with AI for real-time monitoring of intraocular pressure (IOP), retinal health, and vision parameters. These devices can help detect early signs of glaucoma or diabetic retinopathy, enabling timely interventions.
- *Integration with augmented reality (AR):* Combine AI and AR in ophthalmic surgeries to enhance precision. For example, AR could overlay real-time AI-processed images during cataract or retinal surgery, guiding surgeons for improved outcomes.
- *Predictive models for retinal diseases:* Build AI tools to predict the progression of retinal diseases, such as age-related macular degeneration (AMD) based on patient-specific data, enabling preemptive management strategies.

CONCLUSION

Artificial intelligence has revolutionized ophthalmology, providing new tools for early disease detection, accurate diagnostics, surgical planning, and patient monitoring. From detecting DR and glaucoma to planning cataract surgery and supporting postoperative care, AI applications enhance every stage of ophthalmic care. These advancements have led to faster, more accurate, and more personalized treatments, ultimately improving patient outcomes and preserving vision.

As AI technology continues to evolve, it will likely become even more integrated into clinical workflows, empowering ophthalmologists to provide proactive, data-driven care. The future of AI in ophthalmology promises greater precision, personalized interventions, and better quality of life for patients with ocular diseases. By leveraging AI's capabilities, ophthalmologists can stay ahead of complex diseases and deliver exceptional, individualized care that adapts to each patient's unique needs.

Artificial Intelligence in Oncology

INTRODUCTION

The field of oncology has witnessed transformative changes with the integration of artificial intelligence (AI), allowing for significant advancements in cancer detection, diagnosis, staging, treatment planning, and monitoring. AI-driven tools are proving essential in early cancer detection, optimizing personalized treatment approaches, and improving outcomes for patients. In oncology, AI applications span radiology, pathology, genomics, and even chemotherapy dosing, making cancer care more precise, effective, and individualized. This chapter provides an in-depth exploration of AI's role in oncology, focusing on cancer detection, staging, treatment response prediction, and personalized care strategies.

ARTIFICIAL INTELLIGENCE-DRIVEN TOOLS FOR CANCER DETECTION, STAGING, AND PERSONALIZED TREATMENT PLANNING

Artificial intelligence technologies, particularly machine learning and deep learning, have revolutionized cancer detection and diagnosis. These technologies enable clinicians to detect malignancies at earlier stages, classify tumors more accurately, and devise treatment plans tailored to the unique profile of each patient.

Cancer Detection through Imaging

Early cancer detection is crucial in improving survival rates, and AI enhances imaging accuracy in identifying malignancies across different types of cancer, such as lung, breast, and colorectal cancers. By analyzing imaging data, AI can identify abnormalities, assess tumor characteristics, and provide radiologists with decision support.

- *Example application:* AI models analyze mammograms to detect early-stage breast cancer with high sensitivity and specificity, reducing false positives and false negatives, and thus minimizing unnecessary biopsies.
- *Case scenario*: A breast cancer screening center adopts an AI-powered mammography system to detect abnormalities in mammograms. The AI flags subtle signs of cancer in a patient's scan, prompting a follow-up biopsy that confirms an early-stage tumor. The patient receives early treatment, significantly improving her prognosis.

Cancer type	AI detection tool	Outcome
Breast cancer	Mammography analysis	Early detection, reduced false positives
Lung cancer	CT scan analysis	Identification of small nodules, timely intervention

Staging and Tumor Classification

Accurate staging and classification are essential to determine the most appropriate treatment path for cancer patients. AI algorithms help oncologists assess the stage and aggressiveness of tumors by analyzing factors, such as size, location, and the presence of metastases in imaging and pathology data.

- *Example application:* AI tools for magnetic resonance imaging (MRI) and computed tomography (CT) scan analysis assist in classifying tumors based on characteristics, such as size and lymph node involvement, helping oncologists make precise staging assessments.
- *Case scenario*: A patient with a suspected liver tumor undergoes imaging, and an AI tool classifies the tumor as stage II based on its size and lymph node status. The accurate staging allows the oncologist to tailor a treatment plan focused on localized therapies, improving the patient's chances of recovery.

Tumor characteristic	AI role in classification	Outcome
Tumor size, lymph node involvement	Accurate staging	Targeted treatment planning
Metastasis detection	Identification of advanced stages	Personalized care based on disease spread

Personalized Treatment Planning

Artificial intelligence enables precision medicine in oncology by tailoring treatment strategies to the unique molecular and genetic characteristics of a patient's tumor. This approach minimizes unnecessary side effects and increases treatment efficacy by focusing on therapies best suited to the individual.

- *Example application*: AI algorithms analyze genomic data to identify actionable mutations in a patient's cancer, suggesting targeted therapies that are more likely to succeed.
- *Case scenario*: A lung cancer patient's tumor is sequenced, and an AI-driven tool identifies a mutation in the *epidermal growth factor receptor (EGFR)* gene. Based on this finding, the oncologist prescribes a targeted *EGFR* inhibitor, avoiding the need for traditional chemotherapy and improving treatment effectiveness.

Cancer type	AI-driven treatment insight	Outcome
Lung cancer	*EGFR* mutation identification	Personalized therapy, reduced side effects
Melanoma	*BRAF* mutation detection	Targeted treatment with improved outcomes

Predicting Treatment Response and Optimizing Chemotherapy Dosing

One of the most challenging aspects of cancer treatment is predicting how a patient will respond to a given therapy. AI models offer insights into treatment responses by analyzing patient data, genetic markers, and tumor profiles, enabling oncologists to optimize chemotherapy dosing and enhance therapeutic efficacy.

- *Predicting treatment response:* AI algorithms assess a variety of data sources, including genetic information, imaging, and previous treatment outcomes, to predict a patient's response to therapies, such as chemotherapy, immunotherapy, and radiation. This predictive capability helps oncologists select treatments more likely to be effective for individual patients.
- *Example application*: Machine learning models analyze genetic profiles and previous treatment responses to forecast how likely a patient is to respond to immunotherapy, supporting personalized treatment decisions.
- *Case scenario*: A melanoma patient is considered for immunotherapy, and an AI tool analyzes their genetic profile and immune markers to predict a positive response to PD-1 inhibitors. Based on the AI's recommendation, the oncologist prescribes immunotherapy, leading to a favorable outcome with fewer side effects than traditional chemotherapy.

Treatment type	AI prediction role	Outcome
Immunotherapy	Response prediction based on genetic markers	Improved therapy matching
Chemotherapy	Assessing the likelihood of response	Avoidance of ineffective therapies

Chemotherapy Dosing Optimization

Chemotherapy can be a powerful but harsh treatment, often accompanied by severe side effects. AI helps optimize chemotherapy dosing by taking into account a patient's body weight, organ function, genetic makeup, and previous response to treatment, thereby maximizing efficacy while minimizing adverse effects.

- *Example application*: AI models analyze patient-specific factors, such as metabolism and drug tolerance to recommend optimal chemotherapy dosages, reducing the risk of toxicity.
- *Case scenario*: A breast cancer patient requires chemotherapy, and an AI tool calculates an optimal dose based on her renal function and prior treatment responses. The personalized dosing reduces her risk of toxicity, enabling her to complete her treatment with minimal side effects.

Dosing factor	AI optimization role	Outcome
Body weight, organ function	Customized dose recommendation	Reduced side effects, improved treatment adherence
Drug tolerance, genetic markers	Prediction of toxicity risk	Enhanced safety, minimized adverse reactions

Adaptive Therapy and Dose Adjustment

Artificial intelligence supports adaptive therapy, allowing oncologists to adjust treatment doses based on real-time data about tumor response, minimizing drug resistance and improving treatment efficacy.

- *Example application:* AI models analyze tumor response data throughout the course of chemotherapy, suggesting dose adjustments as needed to prevent resistance and optimize outcomes.
- *Case scenario*: A patient undergoing chemotherapy for pancreatic cancer is monitored with AI-driven imaging analysis, which reveals that the tumor is not responding to the initial dose. The AI model recommends a higher dose, which halts tumor progression and improves the overall response.

Adaptation criterion	AI role in dose adjustment	Outcome
Tumor response monitoring	Real-time dose modification	Prevention of drug resistance
Patient side effect tracking	Dose adjustment based on tolerance	Increased safety, better adherence

APPLICATIONS IN RADIOLOGY, PATHOLOGY, AND GENOMICS FOR ONCOLOGY

Artificial intelligence applications in radiology, pathology, and genomics are instrumental in enhancing cancer diagnosis, providing insights into tumor biology, and supporting precision medicine. By integrating AI across these domains, oncologists gain a more comprehensive understanding of each patient's cancer.

Artificial Intelligence in Radiology for Oncology

Radiology is a cornerstone of cancer diagnosis and staging. AI algorithms analyze images from CT, MRI, and positron emission tomography (PET) scans, detecting subtle signs of tumors and helping radiologists identify malignancies earlier than would be possible with human interpretation alone.

- *Example application*: AI-based analysis of lung CT scans identifies nodules that may represent early-stage lung cancer, allowing for prompt intervention.
- *Case scenario*: A high-risk patient undergoes a CT scan, and an AI tool detects a small nodule suggestive of early lung cancer. The radiologist confirms the finding, and the patient begins treatment at an early stage, significantly improving survival odds.

Imaging modality	AI role in radiology	Outcome
CT scan	Nodule detection in lung cancer	Early intervention, improved prognosis
MRI	Tumor boundary delineation	Accurate staging, better treatment planning

Artificial Intelligence in Pathology for Oncology

In pathology, AI-driven image analysis enhances the interpretation of tissue samples, identifying cellular patterns and molecular markers that indicate cancer. AI tools assist pathologists in classifying tumors, grading cancers, and even identifying rare cancers with unique characteristics.

- *Example application:* AI algorithms analyze histopathological slides to identify patterns indicative of specific cancers, such as prostate or breast cancer, reducing diagnostic time and improving accuracy.
- *Case scenario*: An AI system analyzes a biopsy sample from a patient with suspected prostate cancer, identifying cancerous cells and providing a grade for the tumor. This automated grading supports the pathologist in making a timely and accurate diagnosis, leading to prompt treatment initiation.

Pathology application	AI role in analysis	Outcome
Histopathology	Cancer cell identification and grading	Faster, more accurate diagnosis
Molecular marker analysis	Identification of predictive biomarkers	Improved treatment planning

Artificial Intelligence in Genomics for Precision Oncology

Genomic data provides critical insights into cancer biology, revealing mutations that drive tumor growth and informing targeted therapies. AI in genomics helps interpret complex genomic information, identify actionable mutations, and support the development of personalized treatment plans.

- *Example application*: AI-driven genomic analysis identifies mutations in genes like *BRCA*, *EGFR*, and *KRAS*, guiding treatment decisions based on molecular characteristics.
- *Case scenario*: A patient with colorectal cancer undergoes genomic sequencing, and an AI tool detects a *KRAS* mutation that suggests resistance to certain therapies. Based on this insight, the oncologist selects an alternative treatment, increasing the likelihood of a positive response.

Genetic mutation detected	AI application in genomics	Outcome
BRCA mutation	Identification of risk and treatment pathways	Personalized cancer management
KRAS, EGFR mutations	Resistance prediction and drug selection	Improved therapy targeting

FUTURE DIRECTIONS FOR ARTIFICIAL INTELLIGENCE IN ONCOLOGY

- *AI-driven multi-omics analysis:* Integrate genomic, proteomic, and metabolomic data using AI to create comprehensive profiles of cancer patients. This approach will improve precision medicine by identifying optimal therapies based on tumor biology.
- *Real-time radiology and pathology collaboration:* Develop AI systems that enable real-time collaboration between radiologists and pathologists, combining imaging and histological data to refine cancer diagnoses and staging.
- *AI in adaptive immunotherapy:* Implement AI models to predict patient responses to immunotherapies, dynamically adjusting treatment protocols to maximize efficacy and minimize adverse effects.

CONCLUSION

Artificial intelligence has become an invaluable tool in oncology, supporting every stage of cancer care—from early detection and accurate diagnosis to personalized treatment planning and response monitoring. Through applications in radiology, pathology, genomics, and chemotherapy dosing, AI enables oncologists to deliver more precise, effective, and patient-centered care.

Looking forward, AI's role in oncology will continue to grow, with advancements in multiomics, explainable AI, and real-time surgical support paving the way for even greater impact. By integrating AI into oncology practices, clinicians can stay at the forefront of cancer care, improving patient outcomes, reducing mortality, and enhancing the quality of life for cancer patients worldwide.

Artificial Intelligence in Gastroenterology

INTRODUCTION

Gastroenterology, the field focused on the digestive system and its disorders, has seen significant advancements through the integration of artificial intelligence (AI). AI applications in gastroenterology are transforming diagnosis, treatment, and monitoring of gastrointestinal (GI) conditions, particularly in endoscopy, colonoscopy, liver disease, and gut microbiome analysis. AI-driven tools enhance the early detection of GI cancers, identify inflammatory conditions with precision, and utilize predictive analytics for liver disease and microbiome health. This chapter explores the evolving role of AI in gastroenterology, emphasizing its impact on imaging, early diagnosis, and data-driven management of GI disorders.

APPLICATIONS OF ARTIFICIAL INTELLIGENCE IN ENDOSCOPY AND COLONOSCOPY IMAGING

Endoscopic and colonoscopic procedures are essential tools for diagnosing a wide range of GI conditions, including cancers, polyps, and inflammatory diseases. AI-enhanced imaging tools support gastroenterologists by improving visualization, increasing the accuracy of diagnoses, and reducing the potential for missed lesions.

Artificial Intelligence-assisted Polyp Detection in Colonoscopy

Colorectal cancer is one of the most common cancers globally, and its prevention largely depends on the identification and removal of precancerous polyps. AI-powered systems in colonoscopy help detect polyps in real time, reducing the likelihood of missed lesions and enhancing early detection rates.

- *Example application:* Deep learning models trained on thousands of colonoscopy images identify polyps, flagging suspicious regions in real time during the procedure. This aids gastroenterologists in detecting polyps that might be missed by the human eye, especially small or flat lesions.
- *Case scenario:* During a routine screening colonoscopy, an AI-assisted system alerts the gastroenterologist to a small, flat polyp. Thanks to the AI's detection, the polyp is removed, potentially preventing it from developing into cancer.

Polyp type	AI detection role	Outcome
Small, flat polyps	Real-time identification	Reduced risk of missed lesions, early removal
Large or complex polyps	Enhanced visualization	Accurate detection and complete resection

Detection of Barrett's Esophagus in Endoscopy

Barrett's esophagus, a condition that can lead to esophageal cancer, often requires endoscopic screening for early detection. AI algorithms help identify subtle changes in the esophageal lining associated with Barrett's esophagus, aiding in early diagnosis and intervention.

- *Example application:* AI-driven image analysis tools detect areas of abnormal tissue in endoscopic images, highlighting sections of the esophagus with cellular changes indicative of Barrett's esophagus.
- *Case scenario:* An AI-enhanced endoscopy system analyzes images during a procedure on a patient with acid reflux. The system flags sections with potential Barrett's esophagus, prompting the gastroenterologist to perform a biopsy that confirms the diagnosis.

Condition detected	AI application	Outcome
Barrett's esophagus	Early identification of abnormal tissue	Early intervention, reduced cancer risk
Dysplasia in Barrett's patients	Precise biopsy guidance	Improved monitoring and treatment

Detection of Gastrointestinal Bleeding Sources

Endoscopy is often used to locate sources of GI bleeding, which can be life-threatening if left untreated. AI tools analyze endoscopic images to detect bleeding sites, particularly in cases of obscure or small-volume bleeding.

- *Example application:* AI-powered systems highlight areas of active bleeding or subtle lesions during endoscopy, helping gastroenterologists locate bleeding sources more efficiently.
- *Case scenario:* A patient presents with unexplained GI bleeding, and an AI-assisted endoscopy identifies a small ulcer in the duodenum as the bleeding source. The early detection enables the team to treat the ulcer and stop the bleeding, improving patient outcomes.

Bleeding source	AI role in detection	Outcome
Peptic ulcers	Real-time identification during endoscopy	Prompt treatment and bleeding control
Angiodysplasia	Enhanced visualization for small lesions	Reduced risk of rebleeding

EARLY DETECTION OF GASTROINTESTINAL CANCERS AND INFLAMMATORY DISEASES

Early detection of GI cancers, such as colorectal and esophageal cancer, is crucial for improving survival rates. AI tools are enhancing the ability to identify malignancies and inflammatory conditions, such as Crohn's disease and ulcerative colitis at early stages, allowing for more timely and effective treatment.

Artificial Intelligence in Early Detection of Colorectal Cancer

Colorectal cancer screening through colonoscopy is essential for early detection. AI tools that detect and classify polyps as benign or precancerous in real time allow for immediate intervention, significantly reducing the incidence of colorectal cancer.

- *Example application:* AI algorithms analyze colonoscopic images to classify detected polyps, supporting gastroenterologists in distinguishing hyperplastic (benign) from adenomatous (precancerous) polyps.

- *Case scenario:* A patient undergoing screening colonoscopy is found to have a polyp. The AI system classifies the polyp as adenomatous, leading to its immediate removal and potentially preventing future cancer development.

Polyp type	AI classification role	Outcome
Adenomatous polyps	Real-time classification	Precancerous polyps identified and removed
Hyperplastic polyps	Reduced unnecessary biopsies	Improved patient safety, reduced procedures

Artificial Intelligence in Esophageal Cancer Detection

Esophageal cancer often develops from Barrett's esophagus, and early-stage detection is critical. AI systems in endoscopy can detect subtle mucosal changes indicative of early-stage esophageal cancer, improving the likelihood of successful treatment.

- *Example application:* AI-enhanced endoscopic systems analyze high-resolution images to detect suspicious areas in the esophagus, flagging lesions that warrant biopsy.
- *Case scenario:* An AI-powered endoscopy flags a small lesion in the esophagus that appears suspicious. A biopsy confirms early-stage esophageal cancer, allowing for curative treatment and a higher likelihood of survival.

Lesion type	AI role in detection	Outcome
Early-stage esophageal lesions	Real-time detection during endoscopy	Improved survival with early intervention
High-grade dysplasia	Identification of precancerous changes	Timely treatment and monitoring

Detection of Inflammatory Bowel Disease

Inflammatory bowel disease (IBD), including Crohn's disease and ulcerative colitis, requires accurate diagnosis and monitoring for effective management. AI tools analyze endoscopic images to assess the extent and severity of inflammation, supporting treatment decisions.

- *Example application:* Machine learning models evaluate inflammation patterns in endoscopic images, quantifying disease severity in IBD patients and aiding in treatment monitoring.
- *Case scenario:* An AI system assesses inflammation in a Crohn's disease patient's endoscopic images, quantifying the extent of inflammation. The insights help the gastroenterologist adjust the patient's medication to better control disease activity.

IBD type	AI role in assessment	Outcome
Crohn's disease	Inflammation quantification	Optimized treatment plan, disease control
Ulcerative colitis	Severity assessment	Personalized management, reduced symptoms

PREDICTIVE ANALYTICS IN LIVER DISEASE AND GUT MICROBIOME ANALYSIS

Artificial intelligence-driven predictive analytics in gastroenterology extend to managing liver disease and analyzing the gut microbiome. Predictive models assess liver disease progression, predict outcomes, and analyze microbiome composition, enabling personalized interventions and preventive care.

Predicting Liver Disease Progression and Cirrhosis

Liver diseases, such as hepatitis and nonalcoholic fatty liver disease (NAFLD), can progress to cirrhosis and liver cancer if left untreated. AI models analyze patient data, such as liver function tests and fibrosis scores, to predict disease progression and identify high-risk patients.

- *Example application:* AI-based models predict the likelihood of progression from NAFLD to cirrhosis, helping healthcare providers prioritize high-risk patients for close monitoring and lifestyle interventions.
- *Case scenario:* A patient with NAFLD undergoes routine testing, and an AI model assesses the risk of progression to cirrhosis. The system identifies the patient as high-risk, prompting the physician to recommend lifestyle changes and monitor liver function more closely.

Liver disease type	AI prediction role	Outcome
NAFLD	Risk assessment for progression to cirrhosis	Proactive monitoring, lifestyle intervention
Hepatitis	Prediction of fibrosis and liver failure	Early intervention, reduced complications

Early Detection of Liver Cancer (Hepatocellular Carcinoma)

Hepatocellular carcinoma (HCC), a common form of liver cancer, often arises in patients with chronic liver disease. AI models aid in detecting early-stage liver cancer by analyzing imaging and biomarker data, enabling timely intervention.

- *Example application:* AI systems integrate magnetic resonance imaging (MRI) and computed tomography (CT) imaging data with biomarker analysis to detect small, early-stage liver tumors, allowing for curative treatments.
- *Case scenario:* An AI system analyzes MRI scans of a hepatitis patient and detects a small lesion suggestive of early-stage HCC. The early detection allows for immediate treatment, significantly improving the patient's prognosis.

Cancer stage	AI role in detection	Outcome
Early-stage HCC	Identification of small tumors	Improved survival with curative intervention
Advanced HCC	Accurate staging and treatment planning	Optimized therapy based on disease extent

Gut Microbiome Analysis

The gut microbiome plays a vital role in digestive health, immunity, and overall well-being. AI-driven microbiome analysis tools evaluate bacterial composition and diversity, providing insights into conditions, such as IBD, irritable bowel syndrome (IBS), and even metabolic diseases.

- *Example application:* Machine learning models analyze gut microbiome data to identify patterns associated with diseases and predict responses to dietary or probiotic interventions.
- *Case scenario:* A patient with IBS provides a stool sample for microbiome analysis. The AI tool identifies imbalances in bacterial diversity, guiding the gastroenterologist to recommend specific dietary changes and probiotic supplements, leading to symptom improvement.

Microbiome imbalance	AI application in analysis	Outcome
Dysbiosis in IBS	Detection of bacterial imbalance	Personalized dietary and probiotic interventions
Inflammatory patterns in IBD	Prediction of flare-ups	Preventive care and symptom management

FUTURE DIRECTIONS FOR ARTIFICIAL INTELLIGENCE IN GASTROENTEROLOGY

- *AI-enhanced capsule endoscopy:* Use AI to analyze images from capsule endoscopy for detecting gastrointestinal (GI) lesions, polyps, and bleeding sources, reducing reliance on traditional endoscopic methods.
- *Predictive analytics for liver disease:* Develop predictive models for conditions, such as nonalcoholic fatty liver disease (NAFLD) to identify patients at risk of cirrhosis or hepatocellular carcinoma early, enabling targeted interventions.
- *Microbiome-based therapeutics:* Employ AI to study gut microbiome compositions and predict patient responses to dietary changes, probiotics, or fecal microbiota transplants for GI disorders, such as irritable bowel syndrome (IBS).

CONCLUSION

Artificial intelligence has become a critical tool in gastroenterology, enhancing the accuracy, efficiency, and personalization of care for GI diseases. From assisting in polyp detection during colonoscopy and identifying early signs of liver disease to analyzing gut microbiome data, AI applications are transforming every aspect of digestive health management.

Looking ahead, advancements in AI will continue to push the boundaries of what is possible in gastroenterology. By integrating AI into clinical workflows, gastroenterologists can improve diagnostic precision, tailor treatments to individual patients, and proactively manage chronic GI conditions. The future of AI in gastroenterology promises to deliver more accessible, effective, and personalized care for patients, ultimately improving outcomes and quality of life for individuals affected by GI disorders.

Artificial Intelligence in Neurology

INTRODUCTION

Neurology, the field focused on disorders of the nervous system, has seen significant advancements with the integration of artificial intelligence (AI). AI applications in neurology are improving diagnostic accuracy, supporting early intervention, and enabling personalized treatment planning for complex neurological conditions. From neuroimaging and diagnosis of neurodegenerative diseases to stroke detection, epilepsy management, and outcome prediction, AI is revolutionizing neurology. This chapter explores how AI-powered tools are transforming the diagnosis, monitoring, and management of neurological conditions, enhancing the quality of care for patients.

ARTIFICIAL INTELLIGENCE IN NEUROIMAGING AND DIAGNOSIS OF NEURODEGENERATIVE DISEASES

Artificial intelligence's role in neuroimaging has transformed the diagnosis and assessment of neurodegenerative diseases, including Alzheimer's, Parkinson's, and amyotrophic lateral sclerosis (ALS). By analyzing brain imaging data with high precision, AI enables early detection, monitoring of disease progression, and identification of biomarkers that support personalized treatment strategies.

Artificial Intelligence in Alzheimer's Disease Diagnosis and Prognosis

Alzheimer's disease is a progressive neurodegenerative disorder characterized by memory loss and cognitive decline. Early diagnosis and intervention are crucial in managing Alzheimer's, as treatment options are more effective when applied at the early stages. AI models can analyze brain scans, detect biomarkers associated with Alzheimer's, and assess disease progression, allowing for timely diagnosis and intervention.

- *Example application:* Machine learning models process magnetic resonance imaging (MRI) and positron emission tomography (PET) scan data to detect early signs of Alzheimer's, such as hippocampal atrophy and amyloid plaque accumulation, which are often challenging to identify through visual inspection alone.
- *Case scenario:* An elderly patient undergoes an MRI for memory loss evaluation. An AI tool analyzes the scan and detects early signs of hippocampal shrinkage, flagging the likelihood

of Alzheimer's. Based on the AI results, the neurologist recommends cognitive therapies and lifestyle adjustments to slow disease progression.

Imaging biomarker	AI detection role	Outcome
Hippocampal atrophy	Early detection of structural changes	Early intervention and management
Amyloid plaques and tau tangles	Identifies risk of Alzheimer's progression	Targeted treatment planning

Artificial Intelligence in Parkinson's Disease Diagnosis and Monitoring

Parkinson's disease (PD) is characterized by motor and nonmotor symptoms due to dopamine neuron degeneration. AI helps analyze MRI data to detect changes in brain structures associated with Parkinson's, enabling early diagnosis and ongoing monitoring.

- *Example application:* Deep learning models analyze diffusion tensor imaging (DTI) data to detect microstructural changes in brain regions affected by Parkinson's, aiding in diagnosis and monitoring disease progression.
- *Case scenario:* A patient with tremors and rigidity undergoes a DTI scan. The AI model identifies abnormalities in the substantia nigra, suggesting early-stage PD. This leads to early treatment initiation, potentially slowing disease progression.

Brain region analyzed	AI role in diagnosis	Outcome
Substantia nigra	Identifies neurodegenerative changes	Early diagnosis, proactive treatment
Motor cortex and basal ganglia	Monitors disease progression	Adjusted treatment based on disease status

Detection and Monitoring of Amyotrophic Lateral Sclerosis

Amyotrophic lateral sclerosis is a progressive neurodegenerative disorder affecting motor neurons. AI aids in the early detection and monitoring of ALS by analyzing neuroimaging data and motor function metrics to assess disease severity and predict progression.

- *Example application:* AI models analyze MRI data, muscle activity patterns, and voice recordings to identify early ALS symptoms, tracking disease progression over time.
- *Case scenario:* A patient with muscle weakness undergoes neuroimaging and voice analysis. The AI system detects patterns consistent with early ALS, allowing the neurologist to initiate therapies that may slow down motor neuron loss.

Parameter monitored	AI role in detection	Outcome
Motor neuron degeneration	Early detection through imaging	Early intervention and therapy
Voice changes, muscle weakness	Progression tracking	Informed treatment adjustments

APPLICATIONS IN EPILEPSY, STROKE DETECTION, AND PREDICTING NEUROLOGICAL OUTCOMES

Artificial intelligence applications in neurology extend to the management of conditions; such as epilepsy and stroke, where early detection and prediction of outcomes are essential for effective care. AI supports real-time monitoring, early diagnosis, and prediction of patient recovery and long-term outcomes.

Artificial Intelligence in Epilepsy Detection and Management

Epilepsy is a neurological disorder characterized by recurrent seizures. AI-driven tools analyze electroencephalogram (EEG) data to detect seizure patterns, predict seizure onset, and support personalized treatment plans, improving patient safety and quality of life (QoL).

- *Example application:* Machine learning models analyze EEG recordings to detect epileptiform patterns and predict seizure likelihood, helping clinicians adjust treatment accordingly.
- *Case scenario:* An epilepsy patient uses an AI-enabled EEG monitoring device that detects early signs of seizure activity. The device alerts the patient to take preventive measures, reducing seizure impact and improving their QoL.

EEG pattern detected	AI role in detection	Outcome
Epileptiform spikes	Seizure prediction and warning	Increased patient safety and autonomy
Background rhythm abnormalities	Assists in epilepsy diagnosis	Timely treatment initiation

Stroke Detection and Outcome Prediction

Stroke is a medical emergency requiring immediate intervention to minimize brain damage. AI enhances stroke diagnosis through rapid analysis of computed tomography (CT) and MRI scans, identifying ischemic and hemorrhagic strokes with high accuracy. Additionally, AI models predict poststroke recovery, guiding rehabilitation efforts.

- *Example application:* AI algorithms analyze CT scans to detect blockages or bleeding in brain vessels, helping clinicians determine the type of stroke and guide treatment decisions.
- *Case scenario:* A patient with stroke symptoms undergoes a CT scan, which an AI model quickly analyzes, identifying an ischemic stroke. The neurologist administers thrombolytic therapy within the critical time window, improving the patient's chances of recovery.

Stroke type	AI detection role	Outcome
Ischemic stroke	Rapid identification of vessel blockage	Timely intervention, improved outcomes
Hemorrhagic stroke	Detection of brain bleeding	Targeted treatment, minimized brain damage

Predicting Neurological Outcomes in Brain Injury

Patients with traumatic brain injury (TBI) or other neurological injuries face uncertain outcomes. AI tools predict long-term neurological outcomes by analyzing imaging data, patient demographics, and clinical factors, enabling personalized rehabilitation plans.

- *Example application:* AI models assess MRI scans, injury severity, and patient characteristics to predict functional recovery, guiding rehabilitation strategies.
- *Case scenario:* A TBI patient undergoes an MRI scan, and an AI model predicts a high likelihood of functional recovery. Based on this information, the rehabilitation team creates an intensive therapy plan that maximizes the patient's potential for recovery.

Predictive factor	AI role in outcome prediction	Outcome
Injury severity, age	Functional recovery prediction	Tailored rehabilitation approach
Brain tissue damage	Long-term outcome assessment	Personalized care, informed family planning

ARTIFICIAL INTELLIGENCE-POWERED TOOLS FOR MONITORING AND MANAGING NEUROLOGICAL CONDITIONS

Artificial intelligence plays a critical role in monitoring neurological conditions and supporting personalized management. Wearable devices, mobile applications, and data-driven AI models allow for continuous monitoring and dynamic adjustments to treatment plans, enhancing patient autonomy and quality of care.

Wearable Devices for Continuous Monitoring

Wearable devices integrated with AI enable continuous monitoring of neurological symptoms, including tremors, seizures, and motor function, offering real-time insights into disease status and enabling timely interventions.

- *Example application:* Wearables with AI algorithms monitor tremor patterns in PD patients, alerting them to adjust medications or take preventive actions.
- *Case scenario:* A Parkinson's patient wears a smartwatch that monitors tremors. The AI in the device detects worsening tremors and sends an alert to the patient's neurologist, prompting a medication adjustment that improves symptom control.

Symptom monitored	AI role in monitoring	Outcome
Tremors in PD	Real-time monitoring and alerts	Better symptom management, improved QoL
Seizure activity in epilepsy	Continuous tracking and warning	Increased patient safety and autonomy

Mobile Applications for Symptom Tracking and Management

Artificial intelligence-powered mobile apps assist patients in tracking neurological symptoms, medication adherence, and lifestyle factors, enabling personalized care and supporting remote monitoring by healthcare providers.

- *Example application:* An AI-driven mobile app for migraine patients tracks headache triggers and predicts migraine onset, helping users avoid triggers and manage symptoms proactively.
- *Case scenario:* A migraine patient uses an AI app that identifies patterns in headache triggers and predicts episodes. By avoiding identified triggers, the patient reduces the frequency and severity of migraines, enhancing their QoL.

Condition managed	AI role in symptom tracking	Outcome
Migraine headaches	Trigger identification and prediction	Reduced frequency and intensity of headaches
Multiple sclerosis (MS)	Symptom tracking and disease monitoring	Proactive adjustments in care

Artificial Intelligence in Personalized Treatment Adjustments

Artificial intelligence algorithms analyze patient-specific data, such as symptom severity and treatment response, to provide personalized recommendations for medication adjustments or therapy modifications, optimizing care for chronic neurological conditions.

- *Example application:* AI-driven models in MS assess disease progression and suggest medication adjustments based on the patient's latest symptoms and MRI findings.
- *Case scenario:* An MS patient experiences worsening symptoms, prompting an AI system to recommend an updated treatment approach. The neurologist adjusts the patient's medications, slowing disease progression and improving their QoL.

Neurological condition	AI role in treatment adjustment	Outcome
MS	Disease progression assessment	Optimized treatment, slowed progression
Epilepsy	Seizure frequency analysis	Adjusted therapy, improved seizure control

FUTURE DIRECTIONS FOR ARTIFICIAL INTELLIGENCE IN NEUROLOGY

- *Neuroplasticity mapping for rehabilitation:* Leverage AI to analyze brain activity and map neuroplasticity patterns, guiding personalized rehabilitation strategies for stroke and traumatic brain injury patients.
- *AI in early neurodegenerative disease detection:* Enhance the detection of early-stage diseases, such as Alzheimer's and Parkinson's by developing AI tools that analyze subtle brain changes in imaging and cognitive assessments.
- *Real-time seizure prediction and management:* Create wearable AI-enabled devices for continuous monitoring and real-time prediction of seizures in epilepsy patients, improving safety and autonomy.

CONCLUSION

Artificial intelligence has become a transformative force in neurology, enhancing diagnosis, treatment planning, and monitoring for a range of neurological conditions. From early detection of Alzheimer's and PDs to seizure prediction, stroke detection, and personalized treatment adjustments, AI applications are making neurology more precise, data-driven, and personalized.

As AI technology advances, its integration into neurology will continue to evolve, with innovations that promise to improve patient outcomes, reduce disease burden, and empower individuals living with neurological conditions. By embracing AI tools, neurologists can deliver better care, proactively manage disease progression, and ultimately improve the QoL for patients with complex neurological disorders.

Artificial Intelligence in Surgery

INTRODUCTION

Artificial intelligence (AI) is playing an increasingly pivotal role in surgery, transforming how procedures are planned, executed, and followed up. From robotic-assisted surgeries to real-time decision support and predictive analytics for postoperative care, AI enables more precise, efficient, and personalized care. This chapter explores the applications of AI in surgical planning, intraoperative decision-making, and postoperative care, emphasizing how these advancements enhance surgical outcomes and patient safety.

ROBOTIC-ASSISTED SURGERY AND ARTIFICIAL INTELLIGENCE IN SURGICAL PLANNING

Robotic-assisted surgery combines robotics and AI to support minimally invasive procedures, enhancing precision and allowing for intricate tasks beyond human capability. Additionally, AI contributes to surgical planning by analyzing patient-specific data and simulating procedures, which enables surgeons to prepare more thoroughly.

Robotic-assisted Surgery

Artificial intelligence-powered robotic systems provide real-time guidance and precision that improve surgical outcomes, particularly in complex or delicate surgeries. These systems enable minimally invasive approaches, which often reduce recovery times, limit blood loss, and decrease the risk of infection.

- *Example application:* The da Vinci Surgical System, an AI-enhanced robotic system, allows surgeons to perform minimally invasive procedures with advanced precision. The system translates the surgeon's hand movements into smaller, more precise motions within the body.
- *Case scenario:* A patient with prostate cancer undergoes robotic-assisted prostatectomy using the da Vinci system. The robotic arms allow for precise removal of cancerous tissue while sparing surrounding nerves, reducing the risk of complications and enabling a faster recovery.

Procedure	Robotic system role	Outcome
Prostatectomy	Precise removal of cancerous tissue	Reduced complication risk, faster recovery
Hysterectomy	Minimally invasive access	Less blood loss, shorter hospital stay

Artificial Intelligence in Preoperative Planning

Artificial intelligence enhances preoperative planning by analyzing medical imaging, anatomical data, and historical outcomes to create customized surgical plans. AI-driven tools provide surgeons with insights into potential challenges and optimal surgical approaches, based on patient-specific factors.

- *Example application:* AI models analyze magnetic resonance imaging (MRI) and computed tomography (CT) scans to create detailed 3D models of organs and tissues, allowing surgeons to visualize the procedure and anticipate complications.
- *Case scenario:* A patient with a complex brain tumor undergoes preoperative planning aided by AI, which provides a 3D model of the tumor and surrounding structures. The model helps the neurosurgeon plan a safe approach to avoid critical areas, minimizing risks and improving the patient's prognosis.

Surgery type	AI's role in planning	Outcome
Brain tumor resection	3D visualization of tumor and structures	Reduced risk to critical brain areas
Orthopedic joint replacement	Customized implant positioning	Improved fit and longevity of implants

Patient-specific Surgical Simulation

Artificial intelligence simulations provide virtual environments where surgeons can practice complex procedures, reducing risks by familiarizing them with the patient's unique anatomy and potential challenges before the actual surgery.

- *Example application:* Virtual reality (VR) simulators powered by AI allow surgeons to perform "dry runs" of a procedure, using data from the patient's own scans to replicate the specific case.
- *Case scenario:* A cardiac surgeon prepares for a challenging heart valve repair by using an AI-powered simulator that replicates the patient's anatomy based on preoperative imaging. Practicing the procedure in a virtual environment reduces the chance of complications during the actual surgery.

Simulation purpose	AI contribution	Outcome
Complex cardiac procedures	Simulates patient-specific anatomy	Increased surgeon preparedness
Spine surgery	Identifies optimal approach based on anatomy	Reduced intraoperative risks

REAL-TIME DECISION SUPPORT DURING PROCEDURES

Artificial intelligence's real-time decision support capabilities are invaluable in the operating room, where critical decisions need to be made rapidly. AI tools provide intraoperative guidance, alerting surgeons to potential risks and assisting in navigation and precision tasks.

Intraoperative Imaging and Guidance

Artificial intelligence -powered imaging systems provide continuous feedback during surgery, allowing surgeons to see beyond what is visible to the human eye. These systems are particularly useful in guiding complex procedures, such as those involving small structures or critical areas.

- *Example application*: AI-enhanced imaging systems provide real-time analysis of vascular structures during laparoscopic surgery, alerting the surgeon to potential bleeding risks and helping avoid vascular injuries.
- *Case scenario:* During a laparoscopic liver resection, an AI imaging system highlights blood vessels near the target area, reducing the risk of accidental injury. The surgeon adjusts their approach based on AI insights, minimizing blood loss and improving patient safety.

Procedure	AI guidance	Outcome
Laparoscopic liver resection	Identification of vascular structures	Reduced risk of bleeding
Spinal fusion	Real-time imaging of nerve pathways	Avoids nerve damage, reduced postoperative pain

Augmented Reality and Navigation

Augmented reality (AR) in surgery allows AI-generated data to be overlaid onto the surgeon's field of view, providing navigation support and enhancing visualization. This approach helps surgeons maintain accuracy and control, especially in minimally invasive surgeries.

- *Example application:* AR-based navigation systems overlay CT or MRI data onto the patient's body in real time, guiding the surgeon through critical structures and reducing the likelihood of errors.
- *Case scenario:* A spinal surgeon uses an AR system to align screws during spinal fusion surgery. The AI-powered AR system overlays real-time imaging, ensuring the screws are placed accurately and reducing the risk of complications.

Surgery type	AR guidance role	Outcome
Spinal fusion	Accurate screw placement	Reduced risk of misalignment
Tumor excision	Real-time visualization of tumor boundaries	Precise removal, sparing healthy tissue

Artificial Intelligence for Precision Task Assistance

Artificial intelligence can perform or assist with highly precise tasks, such as suturing, excision, and tissue manipulation, allowing surgeons to focus on decision-making rather than manual dexterity. This is especially valuable in surgeries requiring extreme precision, such as ophthalmic and neurosurgical procedures.

- *Example application:* In ophthalmic surgery, AI-driven robots assist with microscopic tasks, such as retinal suturing, by performing steady, precise movements that minimize human error.
- *Case scenario:* An ophthalmic surgeon performs retinal surgery with an AI-assted robotic arm. The AI handles the delicate suturing, reducing the risk of tissue damage and ensuring an optimal outcome for the patient.

Task type	AI role in precision assistance	Outcome
Retinal surgery	Precise suturing of delicate tissues	Reduced risk of complications
Brain surgery	Controlled excision of tumor tissue	Minimal impact on surrounding areas

POSTOPERATIVE CARE OPTIMIZATION THROUGH PREDICTIVE ANALYTICS

Postoperative care is essential for a patient's recovery, and AI-driven predictive analytics can identify potential complications before they arise, allowing for timely interventions and personalized recovery plans.

Predicting Postoperative Complications

Artificial intelligence models analyze patient data to predict the likelihood of complications, such as infection, bleeding, and thromboembolism after surgery. By identifying high-risk patients, healthcare providers can monitor these individuals more closely and take preventive measures.

- *Example application:* AI algorithms use patient demographics, surgical data, and vital signs to predict the risk of postoperative infection, allowing clinicians to intervene proactively.
- *Case scenario:* A patient undergoing abdominal surgery is flagged by an AI tool as being at high risk for postoperative infection based on factors, such as age, body mass index (BMI), and procedure duration. As a result, the care team monitors the patient closely and administers preventive antibiotics, reducing the risk of infection.

Complication type	AI prediction role	Outcome
Postoperative infection	Risk assessment based on patient factors	Early intervention, reduced infection rates
Deep vein thrombosis	Predictive monitoring	Preventive measures, reduced complications

Pain Management and Recovery Tracking

Artificial intelligence-powered tools help track pain levels and recovery metrics, adjusting pain management protocols and identifying issues, such as delayed healing. AI-driven insights into recovery patterns allow for individualized patient care, improving comfort and reducing opioid reliance.

- *Example application:* Machine learning models analyze patient-reported pain scores, vital signs, and healing metrics to recommend personalized pain management adjustments and support faster recovery.
- *Case scenario:* A patient recovering from knee surgery uses a mobile app that tracks pain and mobility levels. The AI in the app suggests adjustments to the pain management plan, reducing discomfort without over-reliance on opioids.

Recovery metric	AI monitoring role	Outcome
Pain levels	Personalized pain management recommendations	Improved comfort, reduced opioid use
Healing progress	Identification of delayed recovery	Adjusted care plan, optimized healing

Readmission Risk Prediction

Hospital readmissions after surgery can signal complications or inadequate recovery support. AI tools predict readmission risks based on patient data, helping healthcare providers implement tailored interventions to reduce readmissions.

- *Example application:* AI models analyze data from surgical procedures, patient demographics, and postoperative progress to identify individuals at high risk for readmission.

- *Case scenario:* An AI tool predicts a high risk of readmission for a patient after cardiac surgery. The care team schedules follow-up appointments and provides home health services, reducing the likelihood of complications that could lead to readmission.

Readmission risk factor	AI role in prediction	Outcome
Postoperative progress	Identification of high-risk patients	Proactive support, reduced readmissions
Medical history	Tailored follow-up and monitoring	Improved recovery, fewer complications

FUTURE DIRECTIONS FOR ARTIFICIAL INTELLIGENCE IN SURGERY

- *Robotic-assisted autonomous surgery:* Develop real-time AI systems for autonomous robotic-assisted surgeries, performing tasks like suturing or lesion removal under surgeon supervision to improve precision and reduce human error.
- *AI-enhanced surgical training simulators:* Build advanced surgical training platforms powered by AI to simulate patient-specific anatomy and surgical scenarios, improving surgeon preparedness for complex procedures.
- *Predictive analytics for postoperative outcomes:* Use AI models to predict risks, such as infections or thromboembolism, enabling proactive postoperative care and reducing complications.

CONCLUSION

Artificial intelligence has revolutionized surgery, bringing new levels of precision, safety, and personalization to the operating room and beyond. From robotic-assisted surgeries to real-time intraoperative guidance and predictive analytics for postoperative care, AI applications are making surgery more efficient and reducing risks for patients.

With continuous advancements, AI's integration in surgery will likely expand further, making procedures less invasive, improving recovery times, and enabling more tailored care. As the field evolves, AI-driven surgical tools and techniques will play a critical role in enhancing patient outcomes, transforming surgical practice, and empowering surgeons to deliver safer, more effective treatments.

CHAPTER 13

Artificial Intelligence in Obstetrics and Gynecology

INTRODUCTION

Artificial intelligence (AI) in gynecology and obstetrics is transforming prenatal screening, fetal monitoring, risk prediction, cancer detection, and reproductive health management. These advancements enhance diagnostic accuracy, improve maternal and fetal health, and allow for early intervention in gynecological cancers. AI-powered tools support clinicians in making data-driven decisions, improving outcomes in prenatal and maternal care, gynecological oncology, and reproductive health. This chapter explores AI's role across these areas, illustrating its impact through real-world applications and case scenarios.

APPLICATIONS IN PRENATAL SCREENING, FETAL MONITORING, AND RISK PREDICTION

Artificial intelligence-driven tools are enhancing prenatal screening, monitoring fetal health, and predicting risks for conditions, such as preeclampsia and preterm birth. These technologies help in identifying potential complications early, allowing for timely interventions that improve maternal and fetal outcomes.

Prenatal Screening and Risk Assessment

Prenatal screening tests are crucial for detecting potential genetic disorders and chromosomal abnormalities early in pregnancy. AI algorithms analyze screening data and genetic information to improve the accuracy of risk assessments, reducing the need for invasive tests and supporting early intervention.

- *Example application:* AI models analyze ultrasound images and blood test results to predict the risk of genetic conditions, such as Down syndrome, Trisomy 18, and neural tube defects with high accuracy.
- *Case scenario:* A pregnant woman undergoes a first-trimester ultrasound and blood screening. An AI system analyzes the data and identifies a high risk for Down syndrome, prompting the healthcare provider to recommend further noninvasive prenatal testing (NIPT) for confirmation.

Condition detected	AI role in screening	Outcome
Down syndrome	Enhanced risk assessment	Timely confirmation through noninvasive testing
Trisomy 18, neural tube defects	Early detection	Improved prenatal planning and management

Fetal Monitoring and Anomaly Detection

Artificial intelligence enhances fetal monitoring by analyzing patterns in fetal heart rate, movement, and growth to detect anomalies. These tools help in identifying signs of fetal distress, growth restrictions, and other conditions that may require early intervention.

- *Example application:* AI-driven fetal monitoring systems analyze data from cardiotocography (CTG) and Doppler ultrasound, identifying patterns that suggest fetal hypoxia or growth restriction, alerting clinicians to potential issues.
- *Case scenario:* A pregnant woman undergoes routine fetal monitoring with an AI-enabled CTG system. The AI identifies signs of fetal distress due to reduced oxygen levels, prompting the healthcare team to schedule an emergency delivery, improving the baby's chances of a healthy outcome.

Fetal condition monitored	AI detection role	Outcome
Fetal hypoxia	Early detection of oxygen deprivation	Timely intervention, reduced risk of complications
Intrauterine growth restriction	Identifies growth abnormalities	Closer monitoring, timely delivery

Risk Prediction for Preeclampsia and Preterm Birth

Preeclampsia and preterm birth are significant complications in pregnancy, often leading to adverse maternal and fetal outcomes. AI tools predict the likelihood of these conditions by analyzing patient data, such as blood pressure, protein levels, and maternal history, allowing for preventive measures.

- *Example application:* Machine learning algorithms analyze maternal health records, including blood pressure and proteinuria, to predict the risk of preeclampsia, supporting early intervention.
- *Case scenario:* An expectant mother's medical records are analyzed by an AI system that predicts a high risk for preeclampsia. Based on this information, her healthcare provider increases monitoring and initiates preventive treatment, reducing the likelihood of severe complications.

Risk factor analyzed	AI prediction role	Outcome
Blood pressure, protein levels	Early prediction of preeclampsia risk	Preventive care, reduced severity
Maternal history, lifestyle factors	Prediction of preterm birth	Timely planning for potential early delivery

ARTIFICIAL INTELLIGENCE FOR EARLY DETECTION AND MANAGEMENT OF GYNECOLOGICAL CANCERS

Artificial intelligence applications in gynecology are instrumental in the early detection and management of gynecological cancers, such as cervical, ovarian, and endometrial cancers. By improving screening accuracy and guiding treatment plans, AI aids in reducing cancer mortality and enhancing patient outcomes.

Cervical Cancer Screening and Detection

Cervical cancer is preventable through regular screening, yet it remains a leading cause of cancer-related deaths in women worldwide. AI tools enhance Pap smear analysis, identifying cellular abnormalities associated with precancerous changes and human papillomavirus (HPV) infection.

- *Example application:* Deep learning models analyze Pap smear and HPV test images, accurately identifying abnormal cells that may indicate cervical cancer or precancerous conditions.
- *Case scenario:* A 35-year-old woman undergoes a routine Pap smear, and the AI-enhanced analysis identifies atypical cells with signs of HPV infection. The early detection prompts a follow-up colposcopy and biopsy, allowing for early treatment and reducing her cancer risk.

Cellular abnormality detected	AI screening role	Outcome
Atypical cells, HPV infection	Early identification of high-risk lesions	Early intervention, reduced cancer risk
Low- and high-grade lesions	Precancerous condition detection	Preventive treatment, improved outcomes

Ovarian Cancer Detection and Prognosis

Ovarian cancer often goes undetected until it is advanced, making early diagnosis critical. AI-driven algorithms analyze imaging and genetic data to identify early-stage ovarian cancer, improving prognosis and treatment planning.

- *Example application:* AI models analyze ultrasound and computed tomography (CT) images to detect small ovarian masses that may indicate early cancer, while also assessing tumor markers in blood tests.
- *Case scenario:* A patient with vague abdominal symptoms undergoes an AI-assisted ultrasound, which detects a suspicious ovarian mass. The AI model recommends additional tests, leading to an early diagnosis of ovarian cancer and timely surgical intervention.

Imaging and biomarker analysis	AI role in detection	Outcome
Ovarian mass identification	Early detection of potential malignancy	Improved prognosis through early surgery
Tumor marker assessment	Risk assessment for ovarian cancer	Guided follow-up and monitoring

Endometrial Cancer Risk Prediction and Management

Endometrial cancer, the most common gynecological cancer, is often diagnosed at an early stage. However, AI can further aid in risk prediction and help customize treatment based on the patient's individual risk profile.

- *Example application:* Machine learning algorithms analyze factors, such as obesity, diabetes, and menstrual history to predict endometrial cancer risk, supporting preventive measures and tailored treatment plans.
- *Case scenario:* An overweight, postmenopausal woman's health data is analyzed by an AI tool that flags her as high risk for endometrial cancer. This prompts her doctor to recommend regular screenings and preventive lifestyle changes, reducing her cancer risk.

Risk factor assessed	AI's role in risk prediction	Outcome
Obesity, diabetes	Identification of high-risk individuals	Preventive screenings, lifestyle modification
Family history, hormonal factors	Prediction of endometrial cancer risk	Early diagnosis, personalized care

ENHANCEMENTS IN REPRODUCTIVE HEALTH AND MATERNAL CARE

Artificial intelligence plays an important role in reproductive health, from fertility treatments to personalized maternal care. AI-powered systems provide insights into menstrual health, fertility, and maternal conditions, supporting women in managing reproductive and maternal health effectively.

Artificial Intelligence in Fertility Treatments

Artificial intelligence enhances fertility treatments by predicting ovulation cycles, selecting optimal embryos for implantation, and customizing treatment plans based on individual patient profiles. This increases the success rates of procedures, such as in vitro fertilization (IVF).

- *Example application:* AI algorithms analyze patient-specific data to predict optimal IVF timing, select viable embryos, and improve implantation success rates.
- *Case scenario:* A woman undergoing IVF receives embryo selection assistance from an AI system that analyzes embryo images. The selected embryo has a higher implantation probability, leading to a successful pregnancy.

Fertility treatment component	AI role in optimization	Outcome
Embryo selection	Identification of viable embryos	Increased IVF success rates
Ovulation timing	Accurate cycle prediction	Improved timing for conception

Personalized Menstrual and Hormonal Health Monitoring

Artificial intelligence-driven apps and wearables track menstrual cycles, hormonal fluctuations, and symptoms, providing personalized insights into reproductive health. These tools help women manage conditions, such as polycystic ovary syndrome (PCOS) and premenstrual syndrome (PMS).

- *Example application:* AI-powered menstrual health apps analyze cycle data to provide predictions for ovulation, fertility windows, and symptom management advice.
- *Case scenario:* A woman with irregular cycles uses an AI-powered app that identifies patterns indicative of PCOS. With this insight, she consults her doctor and begins a management plan, improving her menstrual health.

Health aspect monitored	AI's role in monitoring	Outcome
Menstrual cycle irregularities	Detection of hormonal imbalances	Early diagnosis and management of PCOS
Symptom tracking	Personalized health recommendations	Improved reproductive health management

Maternal Health Monitoring and Support

Artificial intelligence tools support maternal health by monitoring vital signs, predicting risks for gestational diabetes and preeclampsia, and guiding lifestyle modifications. These tools enable early intervention and provide personalized recommendations to improve maternal and fetal health.

- *Example application:* AI systems monitor maternal blood pressure, glucose levels, and weight gain, predicting the risk of gestational diabetes and guiding preventive care.

- *Case scenario:* An AI-powered app monitors a pregnant woman's blood pressure and weight, flagging an elevated risk for gestational diabetes. Based on this alert, her healthcare provider recommends dietary adjustments and closer monitoring.

Maternal health parameter	AI monitoring role	Outcome
Blood pressure, glucose levels	Early prediction of gestational diabetes	Preventive care, reduced complication risk
Weight gain, physical activity	Personalized lifestyle recommendations	Healthier pregnancy outcomes

FUTURE DIRECTIONS FOR ARTIFICIAL INTELLIGENCE IN GYNECOLOGY AND OBSTETRICS

- *AI for real-time labor monitoring:* Create AI tools to continuously monitor maternal and fetal conditions during labor, identifying signs of distress early to guide timely interventions.
- *Personalized fertility treatment planning:* Use AI to analyze patient-specific data, optimizing fertility treatments, such as in vitro fertilization (IVF) through precise embryo selection and hormonal therapy adjustments.
- *AI in predicting pregnancy complications:* Develop predictive models for risks, such as preeclampsia or gestational diabetes based on patient history, biomarkers, and lifestyle factors, enabling preventive care.

CONCLUSION

Artificial intelligence is revolutionizing gynecology and obstetrics, enhancing prenatal screening, fetal monitoring, risk prediction, cancer detection, and reproductive health management. AI-powered tools improve diagnostic accuracy, support early interventions, and personalize care, ultimately benefiting maternal and fetal health outcomes.

With continuous advancements, AI's role in this field is likely to expand, making care more precise, accessible, and personalized. By integrating AI into gynecology and obstetrics, healthcare providers can deliver higher-quality care, reduce complications, and improve the quality of life for women across various stages of life, from fertility to pregnancy and beyond.

Artificial Intelligence in Clinical Pharmacology and Therapeutic Drug Monitoring

INTRODUCTION

Clinical pharmacology and therapeutic drug monitoring (TDM) are critical to effective and safe patient care, especially when managing complex drug regimens or medications with narrow therapeutic indices. The integration of artificial intelligence (AI) in clinical pharmacology is transforming drug interaction analysis, adverse event prediction, dose optimization, and TDM. AI-based predictive models are aiding clinicians in developing patient-specific drug regimens, optimizing drug dosing, and enhancing patient safety through proactive risk management. This chapter explores AI's role in clinical pharmacology, illustrating its application in adverse event prediction, dose optimization, and personalized pharmacokinetics.

ARTIFICIAL INTELLIGENCE IN DRUG INTERACTION ANALYSIS AND ADVERSE EVENT PREDICTION

Drug interactions and adverse events are significant concerns in clinical pharmacology, particularly in patients with polypharmacy or those on high-risk drugs. AI-powered tools help predict potential interactions and adverse events by analyzing vast amounts of clinical and pharmacological data, thereby reducing risks and improving patient outcomes.

Drug Interaction Analysis

Artificial intelligence models analyze multiple sources of data, including drug properties, patient-specific factors, and real-world evidence, to predict drug interactions. By identifying high-risk interactions, these models help clinicians select safer drug combinations and optimize therapy.

- *Example application:* Machine learning algorithms assess the metabolic pathways of drugs to predict interactions that may lead to adverse effects, such as interactions involving cytochrome P450 (CYP450) enzymes.
- *Case scenario:* A patient with hypertension and diabetes is prescribed multiple medications. An AI-driven drug interaction checker alerts the healthcare provider to a potential interaction between the patient's blood pressure medication and a newly prescribed antidiabetic drug, suggesting an alternative to avoid adverse effects.

Interaction type	AI role in detection	Outcome
CYP450 enzyme interactions	Predicts risk of altered drug metabolism	Prevention of adverse reactions
QT interval prolongation	Identifies drugs that affect heart rhythm	Safer drug selection

Adverse Event Prediction

Artificial intelligence models analyze patient history, genetic information, and drug profiles to predict the likelihood of adverse events. These tools enable proactive monitoring and risk mitigation, enhancing patient safety and treatment efficacy.

- *Example application:* AI algorithms assess patient-specific factors, such as genetics, age, and organ function, to predict the likelihood of adverse reactions, such as hepatotoxicity or nephrotoxicity.
- *Case scenario:* A patient is prescribed a new medication known to have a risk of hepatotoxicity. An AI model, analyzing the patient's liver function and genetic predispositions, predicts a high risk of adverse reaction. The healthcare provider adjusts the dose and increases monitoring to ensure patient safety.

Adverse event type	AI prediction role	Outcome
Hepatotoxicity	Predicts risk based on genetic and liver function	Preventive monitoring and dose adjustment
Nephrotoxicity	Assesses risk based on kidney function	Safer dosing, reduced kidney injury

Polypharmacy and High-risk Drug Regimens

In patients with multiple medications, AI helps in managing polypharmacy by identifying potentially harmful drug combinations and recommending safer alternatives. This is especially crucial for elderly patients and those with complex medical histories.

- *Example application:* AI models identify potentially inappropriate medications in polypharmacy, supporting deprescribing efforts to minimize adverse events and improve outcomes.
- *Case scenario:* An elderly patient on multiple medications is evaluated by an AI tool that flags a risky combination of sedatives and antihypertensives, suggesting a safer regimen. This adjustment reduces the risk of falls and other complications related to sedation and blood pressure.

Polypharmacy issue	AI's role in safety management	Outcome
Sedative and antihypertensive combination	Flags high-risk interactions	Reduced fall risk, optimized therapy
Potentially inappropriate drugs	Recommends alternative medications	Improved safety and adherence

DOSE OPTIMIZATION AND THERAPEUTIC DRUG MONITORING

Artificial intelligence's ability to process real-time patient data and analyze complex pharmacokinetic and pharmacodynamic relationships is invaluable in dose optimization and TDM. AI models support precise dose adjustments, particularly for drugs with narrow therapeutic ranges, to enhance treatment efficacy and reduce toxicity.

Individualized Dose Adjustment

Artificial intelligence models analyze patient characteristics, including weight, organ function, and genetics, to recommend individualized doses. This approach is particularly valuable in managing drugs, such as anticoagulants, immunosuppressants, and chemotherapeutic agents, where small dosing errors can lead to serious consequences.

- *Example application:* Machine learning algorithms predict the optimal dose of warfarin based on patient-specific factors, such as age, genetic profile, and concurrent medications, minimizing the risk of bleeding or clotting.
- *Case scenario:* A patient on warfarin therapy has an AI-driven dose calculator that adjusts dosing based on real-time international normalized ratio (INR) levels and genetic factors. This precise dosing reduces the risk of hemorrhage and improves therapeutic efficacy.

Drug type	AI role in dose optimization	Outcome
Anticoagulants (e.g., warfarin)	Dose adjustment based on INR and genetics	Reduced bleeding/clotting risk, safer therapy
Immunosuppressants	Custom dosing to prevent rejection/toxicity	Optimized balance between efficacy and safety

Therapeutic Drug Monitoring

Artificial intelligence-powered TDM tools assist in monitoring drugs with narrow therapeutic indices, such as digoxin, lithium, and certain antibiotics. These tools analyze blood levels and patient factors to recommend dose adjustments, ensuring that drug levels remain within therapeutic ranges.

- *Example application:* AI models integrate patient blood concentration data with pharmacokinetic profiles to recommend dosage changes for drugs, such as vancomycin, optimizing therapeutic levels and minimizing toxicity.
- *Case scenario:* A patient on vancomycin is monitored by an AI system that adjusts dosing based on trough levels and renal function. This personalized TDM reduces the risk of nephrotoxicity while maintaining effective infection control.

Medication monitored	AI's role in TDM	Outcome
Vancomycin	Adjusts dose based on trough levels	Minimized toxicity, effective infection control
Lithium	Maintains therapeutic levels	Reduced risk of lithium toxicity

Managing Drugs with Variable Pharmacodynamics

For drugs with highly variable pharmacodynamic responses, AI models help adjust doses based on real-time feedback from patients' responses to medication. This ensures that the dose is both safe and effective, particularly for drugs with variable effects like insulin.

- *Example application:* AI-driven insulin management systems adjust dosing based on glucose monitoring, physical activity, and dietary intake, providing real-time adjustments to avoid hypo- or hyperglycemia.
- *Case scenario:* A diabetic patient uses an AI-powered insulin pump that adjusts insulin dosing in response to continuous glucose monitoring. The system helps maintain stable glucose levels, reducing the frequency of hypo- and hyperglycemic events.

Variable response drug	AI role in real-time adjustment	Outcome
Insulin	Adjusts dosing based on glucose monitoring	Improved glucose control, reduced hypoglycemia risk
Opioid analgesics	Adjusts dose based on pain levels	Effective pain control, minimized side effects

PREDICTIVE TOOLS FOR PHARMACOKINETICS AND PATIENT-SPECIFIC DRUG REGIMENS

Artificial intelligence tools in pharmacokinetics analyze absorption, distribution, metabolism, and excretion of drugs to predict how individual patients will respond to a specific medication regimen. This enables the creation of patient-specific drug plans, maximizing therapeutic efficacy and minimizing adverse effects.

Pharmacokinetic Modeling for Drug Absorption and Metabolism

Artificial intelligence-based pharmacokinetic models use patient-specific data to predict how drugs will be absorbed, distributed, and metabolized, allowing for tailored drug regimens. This is particularly valuable for medications metabolized by enzymes with genetic variability, like CYP450 enzymes.

- *Example application:* Machine learning models predict how patients will metabolize drugs based on genetic and physiological data, enabling dose adjustments for medications processed by CYP450 enzymes.
- *Case scenario:* A patient prescribed a CYP450-metabolized antidepressant undergoes pharmacogenetic testing, and the AI system tailors the dose based on the patient's metabolism speed. This prevents suboptimal effects due to rapid metabolism.

Drug metabolism type	AI role in metabolism prediction	Outcome
CYP450-metabolized drugs	Predicts metabolism speed	Dose adjustment for optimal therapeutic effect
Drugs with variable absorption	Adjusts dosing based on predicted levels	Improved efficacy, reduced adverse effects

Patient-specific Regimen Design

Artificial intelligence aids in designing drug regimens tailored to each patient's unique physiology and medical history, reducing adverse effects and improving adherence. These systems consider factors, such as weight, age, organ function, and concurrent diseases to develop individualized plans.

- *Example application:* AI-driven models develop customized drug regimens for chronic conditions, such as hypertension and diabetes, accounting for patient-specific factors to enhance efficacy and adherence.
- *Case scenario:* A hypertensive patient with renal impairment is prescribed a personalized regimen developed by an AI model. The regimen considers the patient's kidney function, reducing the risk of drug accumulation and adverse effects.

Patient condition	AI's role in regimen personalization	Outcome
Renal impairment	Customized drug dosing for renal function	Minimized accumulation and toxicity
Chronic diseases (e.g., diabetes)	Dose adjustments for concurrent conditions	Improved adherence, optimized therapy

Predicting Long-term Drug Response

Artificial intelligence can analyze historical patient data to predict long-term responses to medications, supporting proactive adjustments in chronic therapies, such as those for asthma, rheumatoid arthritis, and hypertension.

- *Example application:* AI models use historical treatment data and patient characteristics to predict how long a patient will respond to a particular medication, allowing clinicians to adjust therapy before efficacy declines.
- *Case scenario:* An asthma patient's treatment response data is analyzed by an AI tool that predicts a declining response to current therapy within six months. The clinician proactively switches medications, preventing symptom worsening.

Condition managed	AI role in long-term prediction	Outcome
Asthma	Predicts diminishing response to medication	Proactive therapy adjustment, maintained control
Hypertension	Monitors blood pressure trends over time	Preventive medication adjustments

FUTURE DIRECTIONS FOR ARTIFICIAL INTELLIGENCE IN CLINICAL PHARMACOLOGY AND THERAPEUTIC DRUG MONITORING

- *Multi-omics in drug response prediction:* Integrate genetic, proteomic, and metabolomic data using AI to improve predictions of individual drug responses, enabling more accurate personalized therapies.
- *Real-time dose optimization tools:* Build AI systems that dynamically adjust dosages based on real-time data, such as blood drug levels, vital signs, and patient feedback, ensuring optimal therapeutic effects.
- *Predictive models for polypharmacy management:* Develop AI models to identify and mitigate risks of adverse drug interactions in patients on complex medication regimens, particularly in elderly populations.

CONCLUSION

Artificial intelligence is redefining clinical pharmacology and TDM, enabling personalized drug regimens, optimized dosing, and proactive risk management. From predicting adverse events to adjusting doses for drugs with narrow therapeutic indices, AI supports safer, more effective, and patient-centered pharmacotherapy.

As AI continues to advance, its applications in clinical pharmacology will expand, making treatment regimens increasingly precise and improving outcomes across various patient populations. By leveraging AI, healthcare providers can enhance medication safety, reduce adverse effects, and ultimately deliver more individualized care, ensuring that each patient receives the most appropriate and effective therapy.

Artificial Intelligence in Pediatrics

INTRODUCTION

The integration of artificial intelligence (AI) into pediatrics has brought transformative changes, improving early detection, diagnostics, and personalized care for children. With unique physiological and developmental characteristics, pediatric care requires precision and adaptability, and AI plays a crucial role in achieving these goals. From early disease screening to developmental monitoring and AI-powered diagnostics in neonatal and adolescent health, AI is enhancing pediatric healthcare by enabling early interventions, accurate diagnostics, and tailored treatment plans. This chapter explores the multifaceted applications of AI in pediatrics, highlighting real-world case scenarios and practical implementations.

ARTIFICIAL INTELLIGENCE APPLICATIONS IN EARLY CHILDHOOD DISEASE DETECTION AND SCREENING

Early disease detection is critical in pediatrics, as timely interventions can prevent long-term complications and improve outcomes. AI technologies facilitate screening and early diagnosis for a wide range of childhood diseases, including genetic disorders, congenital anomalies, and infectious diseases, aiding clinicians in providing prompt and effective care.

Screening for Genetic and Congenital Disorders

Artificial intelligence algorithms analyze newborn screening data, genetic information, and imaging to detect congenital abnormalities and genetic disorders at an early stage. By identifying conditions, such as congenital heart defects and metabolic disorders, AI supports early interventions that can significantly improve long-term outcomes.

- *Example application:* Machine learning models analyze newborn screening data, detecting patterns indicative of genetic disorders, such as phenylketonuria (PKU) and congenital hypothyroidism, which may not have immediate symptoms but require prompt treatment.
- *Case scenario:* A newborn is screened for genetic disorders using an AI-enhanced analysis of blood samples. The AI identifies signs of PKU, prompting early dietary management that prevents cognitive impairment.

Condition screened	AI role in detection	Outcome
PKU	Detection through newborn blood analysis	Early dietary intervention, improved cognitive outcomes
Congenital hypothyroidism	Identification via hormonal markers	Timely hormone replacement therapy

Identifying Autism Spectrum Disorder and Developmental Delays

Artificial intelligence tools analyze behavioral patterns, facial expressions, and speech to detect early signs of autism spectrum disorder (ASD) and other developmental delays. These tools facilitate early diagnosis and intervention, which are crucial in optimizing developmental outcomes.

- *Example application:* AI-driven video analysis assesses a child's facial expressions, eye contact, and interaction patterns, identifying behaviors associated with ASD that may go unnoticed in traditional assessments.
- *Case scenario:* Parents of a 2-year-old child notice delays in social interaction. An AI-powered app analyzes videos of the child's behavior, detecting early signs of ASD. This prompts early referral to a developmental specialist, leading to timely intervention with behavioral therapy.

Developmental indicator	AI screening role	Outcome
Eye contact and facial expressions	Early identification of ASD risk	Early intervention with behavioral therapy
Speech and interaction patterns	Detection of social and communication delays	Improved developmental support

Screening for Infectious Diseases in Pediatrics

Artificial intelligence applications in pediatrics support the rapid diagnosis of infectious diseases by analyzing clinical data and laboratory results, improving timely treatment, and reducing the spread of infections in vulnerable pediatric populations.

- *Example application:* Machine learning models analyze symptoms, blood work, and imaging to detect infections, such as pneumonia, meningitis, and sepsis in children, guiding prompt treatment.
- *Case scenario:* An infant presents with fever and lethargy, and an AI-driven tool analyzes clinical data, predicting a high risk of sepsis. The early alert prompts immediate intervention with antibiotics, improving the infant's prognosis.

Infection type	AI detection role	Outcome
Sepsis	Early identification from clinical data	Rapid treatment, improved survival rates
Pneumonia	Risk assessment from imaging and lab results	Timely initiation of appropriate therapy

ENHANCING PEDIATRIC CARE WITH PREDICTIVE TOOLS AND DEVELOPMENTAL MONITORING

Artificial intelligence-powered predictive tools and developmental monitoring applications are enhancing pediatric care by tracking growth, predicting risks, and providing personalized insights into a child's health trajectory. These tools support preventive care and allow for early intervention in developmental issues.

Predictive Tools for Pediatric Growth and Development

Artificial intelligence algorithms track growth patterns, nutrition, and other health metrics to predict growth trajectories, helping identify deviations that may indicate underlying health issues or nutritional deficiencies.

- *Example application:* AI-driven growth charts compare a child's growth metrics to population data, identifying potential deviations in growth rate that could indicate issues, such as growth hormone deficiency.
- *Case scenario:* A young child is monitored for growth, and an AI tool flags that their height growth rate has fallen below expected norms. Early detection leads to further evaluation, diagnosing growth hormone deficiency, and starting treatment to support normal development.

Growth parameter	AI's role in monitoring	Outcome
Height and weight tracking	Early detection of growth delays	Timely intervention, improved growth outcomes
Nutritional status	Predicts deficiencies and recommends supplements	Enhanced nutritional support

Developmental Milestone Monitoring

Artificial intelligence applications monitor developmental milestones, such as motor skills, speech, and social behaviors, allowing for early detection of developmental delays. These tools provide tailored insights to parents and healthcare providers, ensuring timely support and interventions.

- *Example application:* AI-driven apps guide parents in tracking milestones, such as crawling, walking, and speaking, flagging delays that may indicate conditions, such as cerebral palsy or language disorders.
- *Case scenario:* Parents of an infant use an AI-powered app that monitors developmental milestones. When the app detects delayed motor milestones, it suggests consulting a specialist, leading to an early diagnosis of mild cerebral palsy and appropriate therapy.

Milestone monitored	AI role in monitoring	Outcome
Motor milestones	Detects delays in physical development	Early intervention with physical therapy
Speech and language development	Identifies language delay risks	Improved communication skills through therapy

Predictive Modeling for Pediatric Disease Risks

Artificial intelligence models assess genetic and environmental factors to predict the likelihood of pediatric conditions, such as asthma, allergies, and diabetes. By identifying children at high risk, healthcare providers can implement preventive measures and personalized care plans.

- *Example application:* AI tools predict asthma risk by analyzing genetic predispositions, family history, and environmental exposures, guiding preventive measures in high-risk children.
- *Case scenario:* An AI model predicts a high risk of asthma in a young child based on family history and environmental factors. The healthcare provider recommends minimizing exposure to allergens and provides early education on managing potential symptoms.

Condition predicted	AI role in risk prediction	Outcome
Asthma	Identification of high-risk children	Preventive measures, reduced symptom severity
Type 1 diabetes	Predicts genetic predisposition	Early education, monitoring for symptoms

ARTIFICIAL INTELLIGENCE-DRIVEN DIAGNOSTICS AND INTERVENTIONS IN NEONATAL AND ADOLESCENT HEALTH

Artificial intelligence's application in neonatal and adolescent health addresses the unique challenges of diagnosing and managing conditions in newborns and adolescents. AI tools support timely interventions in neonatal intensive care and help manage complex adolescent health issues.

Neonatal Intensive Care Unit Monitoring

Artificial intelligence applications in the neonatal intensive care unit (NICU) analyze vital signs, oxygen levels, and other health data to detect early signs of complications, such as respiratory distress, infections, and cardiac issues, providing critical support in managing high-risk newborns.

- *Example application:* AI-powered monitoring systems in the NICU analyze real-time data to predict complications, such as sepsis or apnea, alerting clinicians to intervene promptly.
- *Case scenario:* A premature infant in the NICU is monitored with an AI-enhanced system that detects patterns suggesting early-onset sepsis. Immediate intervention with antibiotics prevents severe complications, improving the infant's chances of recovery.

Complication monitored	AI monitoring role	Outcome
Sepsis	Early identification from vitals and lab data	Prompt treatment, reduced morbidity
Respiratory distress	Detects signs of breathing difficulties	Early respiratory support, improved outcomes

Mental Health Support and Early Detection in Adolescents

Artificial intelligence tools analyze behavioral patterns, social media activity, and mood indicators to assess mental health risks in adolescents, identifying early signs of anxiety, depression, and other conditions that may require support or intervention.

- *Example application:* AI-driven mental health apps analyze data, such as sleep patterns, social engagement, and self-reported mood to detect mental health risks and recommend resources.
- *Case scenario:* An adolescent using an AI mental health app is flagged for signs of depression based on reduced social interactions and self-reported low mood. The app connects the adolescent with counseling resources, providing early support and preventing symptom escalation.

Mental health indicator	AI's role in detection	Outcome
Social engagement and mood	Early detection of depression risk	Timely mental health support
Sleep patterns and behavior changes	Identification of anxiety indicators	Proactive counseling, symptom management

Management of Chronic Conditions in Adolescents

For adolescents managing chronic conditions, such as diabetes, asthma, or obesity, AI applications provide personalized monitoring and intervention strategies, supporting adherence to treatment, and promoting healthier lifestyles.

- *Example application:* AI-powered apps for diabetes management provide real-time insulin dosing recommendations and track blood glucose levels, helping adolescents manage their condition independently.
- *Case scenario:* An adolescent with type 1 diabetes uses an AI-driven app that monitors blood glucose and provides insulin dosing suggestions based on food intake and physical activity. This support improves glycemic control and empowers the patient to manage their condition effectively.

Chronic condition	AI's role in management	Outcome
Type 1 diabetes	Insulin dosing based on glucose levels	Improved blood sugar control, enhanced independence
Asthma	Monitoring and trigger management	Reduced exacerbations, improved quality of life

FUTURE DIRECTIONS FOR ARTIFICIAL INTELLIGENCE IN PEDIATRICS

- *AI in early childhood neurodevelopment monitoring:* Expand AI applications for tracking motor, cognitive, and language milestones using multimodal data (e.g., video, audio). This can enhance early identification of conditions, such as autism or ADHD and support timely interventions.
- *Personalized pediatric care with genomics:* Leverage AI to integrate genomic data into pediatric care for predicting inherited disorders and tailoring interventions based on a child's unique genetic profile.
- *AI for predictive pediatric population health:* Utilize AI to monitor and predict population-level pediatric health trends, including vaccination compliance and outbreaks of childhood infectious diseases, enabling proactive public health measures.

CONCLUSION

Artificial intelligence is transforming pediatrics, enhancing early disease detection, developmental monitoring, and personalized care in neonatal and adolescent health. From identifying genetic conditions and tracking growth patterns to supporting mental health and managing chronic diseases, AI applications make pediatric care more proactive, precise, and responsive to individual needs.

As AI technology advances, its applications in pediatrics will expand, promising better healthcare outcomes and quality of life for children and adolescents. By integrating AI into pediatric healthcare, clinicians and caregivers can deliver more tailored, timely, and effective interventions, ultimately supporting healthier development and lifelong well-being for young patients.

Artificial Intelligence in Biostatistics for Clinical Practice

INTRODUCTION

Biostatistics is foundational to evidence-based medicine, enabling clinicians to interpret data and make informed decisions. Integrating artificial intelligence (AI) in biostatistics has significantly advanced the ability to analyze complex datasets, predict outcomes, assess treatment efficacy, and support clinical decision-making. This chapter explores the application of AI-driven statistical models in clinical practice, emphasizing how these tools enhance outcome prediction, treatment evaluation, and patient management. Real-world case scenarios and tables illustrate the transformative impact of AI on biostatistical analysis and clinical care.

UNDERSTANDING AND INTERPRETING ARTIFICIAL INTELLIGENCE-BASED STATISTICAL MODELS

Artificial intelligence-based statistical models, including machine learning (ML) and deep learning algorithms, enable the analysis of large, complex datasets. Clinicians need a strong understanding of these models to interpret predictions accurately and make informed treatment decisions.

Types of Artificial Intelligence-based Statistical Models in Clinical Practice

Various AI-based statistical models support different aspects of clinical practice, from predictive modeling to diagnostic classification. Each type has unique strengths and limitations in interpreting and applying data.

- *Logistic regression and decision trees*: These models are frequently used in clinical settings for classification tasks, such as determining the likelihood of a condition based on multiple predictors. Decision trees provide a clear, interpretable pathway, which is valuable for clinicians.
- *Neural networks*: Deep learning models, including neural networks, are useful for analyzing complex, high-dimensional data like medical imaging. However, these models are often less interpretable, which may limit their application in high-stakes decision-making without further explanation mechanisms.

Model type	Clinical application	Strengths
Logistic regression	Risk prediction, binary classification	High interpretability, simplicity
Decision trees	Diagnostic classification	Visual, easy to understand
Neural networks	Image and data pattern recognition	Powerful with large datasets, complex patterns

Interpreting Model Outputs and Uncertainty

Understanding the outputs of AI models is essential, as predictions often come with confidence intervals or uncertainty scores. Clinicians need to interpret these scores to gauge the reliability of a model's prediction and make data-informed decisions.

- *Example application*: In predicting the likelihood of disease progression, an AI model may provide a probability score and a confidence interval. A wider interval may indicate lower model certainty, prompting the clinician to consider additional tests.
- *Case scenario*: A clinician receives a risk prediction for heart disease with a confidence interval of 60–80%. The wide range suggests moderate uncertainty, prompting the clinician to use complementary tests for a more reliable assessment.

Model output	Interpretation in clinical context	Outcome
Probability score with confidence interval	Risk assessment with model certainty	Guides decision on additional diagnostics
Classification score	Indicates likelihood of diagnosis	Supports but does not replace clinical judgment

Addressing the "Black Box" Problem in Artificial Intelligence Models

Many advanced AI models, especially neural networks, operate as "black boxes," meaning that their internal workings are complex and not easily interpretable. Techniques like explainable AI (XAI) help clinicians understand how models reach decisions, enhancing trust in AI-driven insights.

- *Example application*: XAI methods, such as feature importance ranking, highlight which variables (e.g., age and blood pressure) contribute most to a model's prediction, helping clinicians validate the model's reasoning.
- *Case scenario*: An AI model predicts high stroke risk based largely on age and blood pressure. By understanding the model's emphasis on these features, the clinician confirms the model's validity and uses the insight to prioritize preventive measures.

Explainability tool	Role in model interpretation	Outcome
Feature importance ranking	Identifies key variables in prediction	Enhances clinician confidence in AI results
Local interpretable model-agnostic explanations (LIME)	Simplifies complex models for understanding	Supports transparent decision-making

ARTIFICIAL INTELLIGENCE FOR OUTCOME PREDICTION AND TREATMENT EFFICACY IN CLINICAL TRIALS

Artificial intelligence-enhanced statistical models are increasingly used in clinical trials to predict patient outcomes, evaluate treatment efficacy, and identify potential responders. By analyzing diverse datasets, AI supports personalized medicine approaches and enhances clinical trial efficiency.

Outcome Prediction in Clinical Trials

Artificial intelligence models assess patient-specific data to predict outcomes, helping identify patients who may benefit most from a particular treatment. These models consider factors like demographics, genetics, and comorbidities to generate personalized predictions.

- *Example application*: ML models predict individual response to a new cancer therapy by analyzing patient characteristics and historical response data, helping clinicians match patients with the most promising treatments.
- *Case scenario*: A cancer patient's characteristics are analyzed by an AI tool, which predicts a high probability of response to a novel therapy. This information supports the clinician's decision to enroll the patient in the clinical trial, enhancing personalized treatment.

Clinical trial parameter	AI role in outcome prediction	Outcome
Response to cancer therapy	Predicts individual likelihood of success	Informed patient selection, optimized trial outcomes
Risk of adverse effects	Identifies high-risk patients	Preventive measures for patient safety

Evaluating Treatment Efficacy with Artificial Intelligence Models

Artificial intelligence models analyze trial data to assess treatment efficacy, identifying patterns and trends in patient response. This analysis supports faster decision-making in trials and helps determine if a treatment is effective across diverse patient populations.

- *Example application*: Deep learning models assess real-time data from clinical trials, analyzing trends to determine if a drug shows statistically significant efficacy earlier than conventional methods would allow.
- *Case scenario*: In a clinical trial for a new hypertension drug, an AI model identifies an early trend of efficacy in lowering blood pressure. This accelerates decision-making for the trial, potentially speeding up the approval process.

Efficacy indicator	AI role in efficacy assessment	Outcome
Blood pressure reduction	Early trend identification	Accelerated approval for effective drugs
Symptom improvement	Tracks efficacy across subgroups	Tailored analysis for diverse populations

Identifying Potential Responders and Nonresponders

Artificial intelligence models analyze patient data to identify likely responders and nonresponders, enabling more precise patient selection in clinical trials and improving overall trial efficiency.

- *Example application*: ML algorithms analyze genetic data, comorbidities, and treatment history to classify patients by the likelihood of response to a therapy.
- *Case scenario*: An AI tool used in a clinical trial for asthma medication classifies patients based on their genetic profiles, identifying those more likely to respond to the treatment. This targeted recruitment improves trial success rates and optimizes resources.

Responder group	AI prediction role	Outcome
Genetic markers for drug response	Identifies optimal candidates	Higher efficacy rates, reduced trial duration
Comorbidity-based classification	Excludes likely nonresponders	Improved resource allocation, efficient trials

STATISTICAL MODELING FOR PATIENT MANAGEMENT AND DECISION-MAKING

Artificial intelligence-driven statistical models support patient management by providing real-time insights into disease progression, predicting clinical outcomes, and aiding in therapeutic decision-making. These tools help clinicians make personalized, data-driven decisions for optimal patient care.

Predictive Modeling for Disease Progression

Artificial intelligence models predict the likelihood of disease progression, enabling proactive management strategies and personalized treatment adjustments for patients with chronic conditions.

- *Example application*: AI algorithms analyze patient data to predict the progression of chronic diseases like diabetes and heart failure, helping clinicians adjust treatments accordingly.
- *Case scenario*: A diabetic patient's historical glucose data is analyzed by an AI model that predicts worsening control over the next six months. The clinician adjusts the treatment plan, emphasizing lifestyle changes and medication adjustments to prevent complications.

Disease monitored	AI role in progression prediction	Outcome
Diabetes	Predicts worsening glucose control	Proactive treatment adjustments
Heart failure	Forecasts risk of exacerbation	Early intervention, hospitalization prevention

Risk Stratification for Patient Management

Risk stratification models classify patients based on their likelihood of adverse outcomes, allowing clinicians to allocate resources more effectively and prioritize high-risk patients for monitoring or intervention.

- *Example application*: AI models assess patient demographics, comorbidities, and laboratory results to classify patients into risk categories for conditions like stroke, heart attack, and kidney failure.
- *Case scenario*: A healthcare provider uses an AI risk stratification tool that identifies a high risk of stroke for an elderly patient with hypertension and atrial fibrillation. This insight prompts closer monitoring and the addition of preventive medication.

Condition stratified	AI role in risk classification	Outcome
Stroke in atrial fibrillation	Prioritizes patients for preventive care	Reduced stroke incidence, proactive treatment
Kidney failure in diabetes	Flags high-risk patients for monitoring	Improved patient outcomes, targeted interventions

Decision Support for Therapeutic Choices

Artificial intelligence-based decision support systems integrate patient data with clinical guidelines and recent research to recommend personalized therapeutic options, ensuring evidence-based and individualized patient management.

- *Example application*: AI systems that combine data on patient history, laboratory results, and clinical guidelines recommend personalized treatment plans, such as for managing hypertension or cancer.
- *Case scenario*: A patient with hypertension and diabetes receives personalized treatment recommendations from an AI tool that integrates clinical guidelines with his health data. The recommendations guide the clinician in adjusting medication and lifestyle interventions to optimize blood pressure control.

Therapeutic area	AI role in decision support	Outcome
Hypertension management	Recommends optimal drug combination	Improved blood pressure control, personalized care
Cancer treatment selection	Suggests targeted therapies based on biomarkers	Enhanced treatment efficacy, reduced side effects

FUTURE DIRECTIONS FOR ARTIFICIAL INTELLIGENCE IN BIOSTATISTICS FOR CLINICAL PRACTICE

- *Dynamic data integration in real-time analytics:* Develop AI systems that integrate live data from electronic health records (EHRs), wearable devices, and imaging modalities for real-time biostatistical analysis, enhancing decision-making during critical care.
- *Explainable AI models for statistical predictions:* Advance explainability in statistical models to provide clinicians with interpretable and actionable insights, increasing trust and reliability in predictive tools.
- *AI-enhanced adaptive clinical trials:* Design AI systems that dynamically modify trial parameters (e.g., sample size, inclusion criteria) based on interim results, accelerating drug development and improving resource efficiency.

CONCLUSION

Artificial intelligence in biostatistics is redefining clinical practice, offering advanced statistical models that support accurate outcome prediction, treatment efficacy evaluation, and personalized patient management. By leveraging AI-driven insights, clinicians can enhance their decision-making process, make proactive interventions, and improve patient outcomes.

As AI technology continues to evolve, its integration into biostatistics will play a central role in shaping evidence-based, data-driven medicine. The future of AI in biostatistics holds immense potential for making healthcare more precise, efficient, and patient-centered, ultimately contributing to a higher standard of clinical care.

Population Health Management with Artificial Intelligence

INTRODUCTION

Population health management (PHM) is an approach aimed at improving health outcomes for specific populations by addressing broad health issues and promoting preventive care. Artificial intelligence (AI) is transforming PHM by enabling predictive analytics, risk stratification, and targeted interventions for public health and chronic disease management. AI's ability to analyze large datasets and uncover patterns provides valuable insights that support proactive healthcare strategies. This chapter explores the applications of AI in PHM, emphasizing predictive analytics, patient stratification, and interventions that improve public health outcomes and manage chronic diseases.

PREDICTIVE ANALYTICS IN PUBLIC HEALTH AND CHRONIC DISEASE MANAGEMENT

Predictive analytics plays a central role in PHM by identifying trends, anticipating health risks, and enabling early interventions. By applying AI algorithms to population data, healthcare systems can predict disease outbreaks, manage chronic conditions, and develop targeted strategies to improve public health.

Disease Surveillance and Outbreak Prediction

Artificial intelligence-driven predictive models analyze epidemiological data to monitor disease patterns and predict potential outbreaks. By detecting early signs of disease spread, public health agencies can respond promptly to contain outbreaks and prevent widespread health crises.

- *Example application*: Machine learning models analyze data from various sources, such as social media, healthcare records, and environmental data, to detect early indicators of influenza outbreaks and provide timely alerts to healthcare providers.
- *Case scenario*: An AI system monitors social media posts, emergency room visits, and weather data, detecting a sudden increase in flu-like symptoms in a region. The model predicts a flu outbreak, prompting local health authorities to initiate vaccination campaigns and public health warnings.

Disease monitored	AI role in prediction	Outcome
Influenza	Early detection of outbreak signs	Proactive vaccination campaigns, containment
COVID-19	Predicts case surges based on trends	Informed lockdowns, resource allocation

Chronic Disease Management and Progression Prediction

Chronic diseases, such as diabetes, heart disease, and chronic obstructive pulmonary disease (COPD) require continuous management to prevent complications. AI models help predict disease progression by analyzing risk factors and patient history, allowing for timely interventions that reduce hospitalizations and improve quality of life.

- *Example application*: Predictive models analyze patient records to forecast the progression of diabetes, identifying patients at risk of complications like neuropathy or kidney disease and prompting preventive measures.
- *Case scenario*: A diabetic patient's data including blood glucose levels, lifestyle factors, and genetic information is analyzed by an AI model, which predicts a high risk of neuropathy. This prediction enables the healthcare team to implement preventive strategies, such as lifestyle counseling and medication adjustments.

Chronic disease	AI prediction role	Outcome
Diabetes	Predicts risk of complications	Preventive interventions, reduced hospitalizations
COPD	Forecasts exacerbation episodes	Proactive treatment, improved disease control

Predictive Analytics for Resource Allocation in Public Health

Artificial intelligence-driven predictive analytics also aids in optimizing resource allocation by forecasting healthcare demand. By anticipating patient volumes, public health agencies, and hospitals can allocate resources more efficiently, ensuring adequate staffing, supplies, and emergency preparedness.

- *Example application*: AI models predict seasonal surges in hospital admissions, helping healthcare systems prepare by securing additional resources, and optimizing staff schedules.
- *Case scenario*: An AI system forecasts an increase in emergency room visits due to heat-related illnesses during a heatwave. This prediction enables hospitals to increase staffing and prepare cooling resources, minimizing delays and improving patient care.

Public health need	AI role in resource prediction	Outcome
Emergency room demand	Predicts seasonal surges	Optimized resource allocation, improved patient care
Vaccination supplies	Forecasts demand based on population data	Reduced shortages, efficient distribution

APPLICATIONS FOR PATIENT STRATIFICATION AND TARGETED INTERVENTIONS

Artificial intelligence-based patient stratification allows healthcare systems to categorize populations based on health risks, enabling targeted interventions for high-risk groups. Stratifying patients by health risk improves preventive care and ensures that resources are focused where they are most needed.

Risk Stratification for Chronic Disease Management

Risk stratification models categorize patients based on their likelihood of developing or worsening chronic diseases. By identifying high-risk individuals, healthcare providers can offer personalized interventions, reducing hospital admissions, and improving patient outcomes.

- *Example application*: AI models classify patients with cardiovascular disease into risk groups based on factors like age, lifestyle, and medical history, enabling targeted care for those most at risk of heart attacks or stroke.
- *Case scenario*: A health system uses an AI model to stratify heart disease patients by risk of heart attack. High-risk patients receive more intensive monitoring and lifestyle interventions, reducing their likelihood of adverse outcomes.

Condition stratified	AI role in risk classification	Outcome
Heart disease	Identifies high-risk individuals	Focused preventive measures, reduced cardiac events
Type 2 diabetes	Flags patients at high risk of complications	Personalized care, improved disease management

Targeted Interventions for At-risk Populations

Artificial intelligence supports targeted public health interventions by identifying at-risk populations based on demographic, socioeconomic, and health data. These interventions improve health outcomes for vulnerable groups, addressing disparities in healthcare access and quality.

- *Example application*: AI algorithms analyze data on social determinants of health to identify communities at higher risk of conditions, such as obesity and diabetes, guiding targeted nutrition, and fitness programs.
- *Case scenario*: An AI-driven public health initiative identifies neighborhoods with high obesity rates. In response, the local government implements community fitness programs and subsidizes healthy food options, promoting healthier lifestyles and reducing obesity rates.

Targeted health concern	AI role in identifying risk groups	Outcome
Obesity	Identifies high-risk communities	Focused public health campaigns, improved diet, and exercise
Hypertension	Pinpoints areas with high prevalence	Community-based screening and prevention

Early Detection and Proactive Management of High-risk Conditions

Artificial intelligence models help detect high-risk conditions early by analyzing multiple risk factors and biomarkers. Early identification enables proactive management, reducing the burden of disease progression and enhancing the quality of life for affected individuals.

- *Example application*: AI models that analyze biomarkers, genetics, and lifestyle factors predict the onset of Alzheimer's disease years before symptoms appear, supporting early intervention strategies.
- *Case scenario*: An AI tool identifies an individual at high risk for Alzheimer's based on family history and lifestyle factors. This early detection prompts lifestyle modifications and cognitive training that may delay disease onset.

High-risk condition	AI role in early detection	Outcome
Alzheimer's disease	Predicts risk before symptom onset	Preventive lifestyle interventions
Hypertension	Early identification in the prehypertensive stage	Lifestyle adjustments, reduced disease progression

ENHANCING POPULATION HEALTH THROUGH ARTIFICIAL INTELLIGENCE-DRIVEN INTERVENTIONS

Artificial intelligence applications in PHM go beyond prediction, enabling targeted, data-driven interventions that improve population health outcomes. By focusing on specific populations and optimizing interventions, AI supports preventive care and proactive disease management.

Optimizing Preventive Care with Predictive Insights

Predictive insights from AI models allow healthcare systems to optimize preventive care, focusing on vaccination, screenings, and other interventions for at-risk populations. This proactive approach reduces the incidence of preventable diseases and improves long-term health outcomes.

- *Example application*: AI predicts which populations are at risk of low vaccination rates, enabling targeted outreach and education to increase immunization coverage.
- *Case scenario*: An AI tool identifies neighborhoods with low vaccination rates for measles. Public health agencies use this data to conduct targeted outreach, improving vaccination rates and preventing an outbreak.

Preventive care focus	AI role in targeting	Outcome
Vaccination	Identifies areas with low coverage	Increased immunization, reduced outbreak risk
Cancer screening	Predicts the need for targeted mammography campaigns	Higher screening rates, earlier detection

Artificial Intelligence-driven Health Education and Behavior Change Programs

Artificial intelligence helps tailor health education programs to specific populations, promoting healthy behaviors, and reducing risk factors associated with chronic diseases. AI-driven programs improve engagement by personalizing content based on individual preferences and health needs.

- *Example application*: AI-powered apps provide personalized health education, reminding users to engage in physical activity, eat healthily, and adhere to medication, supporting behavior change.
- *Case scenario*: An AI app promotes healthy lifestyle changes in a population with high rates of diabetes. Users receive tailored reminders for exercise and nutrition, leading to improved physical activity levels and better management of blood sugar.

Health behavior targeted	AI role in personalization	Outcome
Physical activity	Tailored reminders and motivation	Increased exercise adherence, improved health
Nutrition	Personalized dietary suggestions	Healthier eating habits, reduced disease risk

Support for Mental Health Interventions and Monitoring

Artificial intelligence supports mental health initiatives by identifying at-risk individuals, monitoring symptoms, and offering timely interventions. These tools improve mental health care accessibility and support early intervention for conditions, such as depression and anxiety.

- *Example application*: AI models analyze social media, language use, and online behavior to detect signs of mental health struggles, prompting outreach and support.
- *Case scenario*: An AI system detects signs of depression in an adolescent's social media activity, alerting mental health providers who offer counseling resources. This proactive approach improves early intervention and mental health outcomes.

Mental health issues addressed	AI role in early detection	Outcome
Depression	Identifies early signs in social media activity	Timely support and counseling, improved outcomes
Anxiety	Detects high-risk individuals through behavior analysis	Early intervention, symptom management

FUTURE DIRECTIONS FOR ARTIFICIAL INTELLIGENCE IN POPULATION HEALTH MANAGEMENT

- *AI in environmental health monitoring:* Incorporate environmental data (e.g., pollution levels, climate factors) into AI models to predict community health risks, particularly for respiratory and cardiovascular conditions.
- *Equity-focused AI for public health:* Develop AI tools that identify healthcare disparities and recommend strategies to bridge gaps in access and outcomes, particularly for under served populations.
- *AI for behavioral health in populations:* Use AI to analyze population-level behavioral data (e.g., social media, wearable metrics) to detect mental health trends, enabling large-scale preventive mental health interventions.

CONCLUSION

Artificial intelligence is revolutionizing population health management by enabling predictive analytics, patient stratification, and targeted interventions. These tools support proactive, data-driven public health strategies that enhance prevention, optimize resource allocation, and improve outcomes for at-risk populations.

As AI continues to evolve, its integration into PHM will transform healthcare delivery, making it more efficient, personalized, and effective. The future of AI in population health promises advancements that not only improve public health outcomes but also promote equity and accessibility, ensuring that all populations benefit from the latest innovations in healthcare.

18

Artificial Intelligence in Enhancing Patient Education and Engagement

INTRODUCTION

Patient education and engagement are essential components of effective healthcare. Educated and engaged patients are more likely to adhere to treatment plans, make informed decisions, and actively participate in managing their health. Artificial intelligence (AI) is transforming patient education by providing personalized tools, improving adherence, and enhancing healthcare literacy. This chapter explores AI's role in delivering tailored health education, fostering patient empowerment, and supporting healthcare literacy. Through practical applications and case scenarios, we illustrate how AI-driven technologies contribute to better health outcomes by enhancing patient knowledge, engagement, and adherence.

PERSONALIZED EDUCATION TOOLS AND PATIENT ADHERENCE IMPROVEMENT

Personalized patient education is key to improving adherence and achieving better health outcomes. AI tools enable tailored information delivery based on individual patient profiles, learning preferences, and health needs, making education more relevant and effective.

Artificial Intelligence-powered Health Education Platforms

Artificial intelligence-powered health education platforms deliver customized information to patients, adjusting the content based on their specific conditions, literacy levels, and learning preferences. These platforms provide interactive resources like videos, quizzes, and real-time feedback to improve patient understanding and retention.

- *Example application*: AI algorithms personalize content for patients with chronic conditions, such as diabetes, by providing information on diet, exercise, and medication management that is tailored to each patient's specific health status and lifestyle.
- *Case scenario*: A patient newly diagnosed with diabetes uses an AI-powered app that provides tailored educational content on blood sugar monitoring, diet management, and insulin use. The content is customized based on the patient's age, literacy level, and lifestyle preferences, making it easier for the patient to understand and implement the advice.

Condition	AI role in education	Outcome
Diabetes	Personalized content on diet and monitoring	Improved patient understanding, better self-management
Hypertension	Tailored education on lifestyle adjustments	Increased adherence to lifestyle changes

Interactive Virtual Health Assistants

Artificial intelligence-driven virtual health assistants offer 24/7 support, answering patient questions, clarifying medical instructions, and providing reminders for medications and appointments. These interactive tools help patients stay informed and engaged in their care by offering guidance in real time.

- *Example application*: Virtual assistants use natural language processing (NLP) to respond to patient queries about medications, procedures, or symptoms, delivering timely information and helping patients feel more supported in their care journey.
- *Case scenario*: A cancer patient uses a virtual assistant that answers questions about chemotherapy side effects and suggests coping strategies. The assistant also reminds the patient to take antinausea medication, improving adherence to supportive care measures.

Use case	AI role in patient engagement	Outcome
Cancer treatment support	Real-time answers and reminders	Reduced anxiety, improved symptom management
Postsurgery care	Guidance on wound care and exercises	Enhanced recovery, better adherence to care plans

Behavioral Nudges and Reminders for Adherence

Artificial intelligence systems provide reminders and behavioral nudges to support medication adherence and lifestyle modifications. These reminders are tailored based on patient-specific factors like medication timing, daily routines, and previous adherence patterns.

- *Example application*: Machine learning models analyze a patient's history and habits to send reminders that align with the patient's routine, making adherence to medication and lifestyle changes easier.
- *Case scenario*: A patient with hypertension receives personalized reminders to take their medication every morning. The AI-driven reminders are scheduled based on the patient's routine, leading to better adherence and improved blood pressure control.

Behavior monitored	AI role in adherence improvement	Outcome
Medication adherence	Timely reminders based on routine	Higher medication adherence, improved health outcomes
Physical activity	Encouragement based on activity patterns	Increased exercise, better disease management

ROLE OF ARTIFICIAL INTELLIGENCE IN PATIENT EMPOWERMENT AND HEALTHCARE LITERACY

Artificial intelligence plays a significant role in empowering patients by providing access to personalized information and supporting healthcare literacy. Empowered patients are better equipped to make informed decisions and actively participate in their healthcare journey.

Personalized Health Literacy Assessments and Education

Artificial intelligence tools assess patients' health literacy levels and tailor educational materials accordingly. By providing information that matches each patient's literacy level, AI promotes better comprehension and engagement, ensuring that patients have the knowledge needed to make informed decisions.

- *Example application*: AI systems assess patients' literacy levels using data on reading comprehension and prior knowledge, delivering information in simple language, or with visual aids as needed.
- *Case scenario*: A patient with limited health literacy is provided with easy-to-understand materials about managing heart failure. The AI system adjusts the content to a simpler language level and includes videos and diagrams to enhance comprehension.

Health literacy level	AI role in tailoring education	Outcome
Low literacy	Simplified content with visual aids	Improved understanding, increased engagement
High literacy	Detailed content with technical terms	Enhanced patient confidence, informed decision-making

Access to Evidence-based Information and Decision Support

Artificial intelligence-driven platforms provide patients with evidence-based information, helping them understand treatment options and potential outcomes. This access empowers patients to discuss options with their healthcare providers and make decisions aligned with their preferences and values.

- *Example application*: AI tools provide summaries of the latest research and treatment options for specific conditions, helping patients weigh the pros and cons of each option with their healthcare team.
- *Case scenario*: A patient with prostate cancer uses an AI-powered platform to learn about treatment options, including surgery, radiation, and active surveillance. The platform presents evidence-based pros and cons for each approach, empowering the patient to make an informed choice in consultation with their doctor.

Condition	AI role in providing information	Outcome
Prostate cancer	Summarizes treatment options	Empowered decision-making, improved satisfaction
Rheumatoid arthritis	Provides evidence on medication efficacy	Informed choice of therapy, better adherence

Patient Engagement through Gamification and Interactive Learning

Gamification and interactive learning modules are effective ways to engage patients and make health education enjoyable. AI can personalize these experiences by adjusting difficulty levels and offering rewards based on patient progress, enhancing motivation and retention of information.

- *Example application*: AI-powered apps create interactive quizzes and challenges related to health topics, rewarding patients for completing tasks and helping them track their learning progress.
- *Case scenario*: A young patient with asthma uses a gamified app that offers quizzes on asthma management, such as recognizing triggers and using inhalers correctly. The app awards points for correct answers, making learning fun and increasing the patient's engagement in self-care.

Health topic	AI role in gamification	Outcome
Asthma management	Interactive quizzes and rewards	Improved self-care knowledge, better adherence to management
Diabetes education	Challenges for tracking blood glucose	Increased awareness of self-monitoring

FUTURE DIRECTIONS FOR ARTIFICIAL INTELLIGENCE IN PATIENT EDUCATION AND ENGAGEMENT

- *AI-driven multilingual health education platforms:* Create multilingual, culturally sensitive AI tools to deliver personalized health education, ensuring accessibility for diverse patient populations globally.
- *Gamification in patient learning:* Expand gamified AI systems for chronic disease management education, promoting patient engagement through interactive learning modules with rewards for compliance.
- *Integration of AI with wearables for real-time education:* Use AI to provide instant feedback via wearables, offering insights on physical activity, nutrition, and medication adherence, thereby reinforcing education in daily activities.

CONCLUSION

Artificial intelligence is transforming patient education and engagement, offering personalized tools that enhance adherence, empower patients, and support lifelong healthcare literacy. By leveraging AI to deliver tailored health information, interactive learning experiences, and real-time support, healthcare systems can improve patient knowledge, foster active participation in care, and ultimately enhance health outcomes.

As AI continues to evolve, its applications in patient education and engagement will become even more sophisticated, providing patients with the resources they need to make informed decisions and take control of their health journey. The future of AI in patient education promises a more empowered, informed, and engaged patient population, contributing to a more collaborative and effective healthcare system.

Legal, Ethical, and Regulatory Considerations for Artificial Intelligence in Healthcare

INTRODUCTION

The integration of artificial intelligence (AI) into healthcare offers transformative possibilities, enhancing diagnostics, treatment planning, patient engagement, and health outcomes. However, the deployment of AI in healthcare also raises significant legal, ethical, and regulatory concerns. Key issues include data privacy, potential biases in AI algorithms, patient consent, accountability, and compliance with regulatory standards. This chapter explores the critical legal and ethical considerations of implementing AI in healthcare, providing an overview of privacy challenges, bias mitigation, ethical guidelines, and the regulatory frameworks designed to ensure safe and responsible AI usage.

Addressing Privacy, Bias, and Ethical Issues in Artificial Intelligence Deployment

Ensuring privacy, minimizing bias, and addressing ethical implications are essential for the responsible implementation of AI in healthcare. These issues have a profound impact on patient trust, data security, and the effectiveness of AI-driven interventions.

Privacy and Data Security in AI-driven Healthcare

Patient data privacy is a fundamental concern in healthcare, and AI applications require extensive data sets to function effectively. Protecting the confidentiality and security of patient information is crucial to maintaining trust and complying with privacy regulations, such as the Health Insurance Portability and Accountability Act (HIPAA) in the United States and the General Data Protection Regulation (GDPR) in Europe.

- *Data anonymization and deidentification:* AI models are often trained on large data sets that include sensitive health information. Data anonymization techniques remove identifiable information, protecting patient privacy while allowing AI to analyze trends across populations.
- *Example application:* Machine learning models analyzing deidentified data from patient records to predict disease trends without revealing individual identities.
- *Case scenario:* A healthcare organization uses deidentified patient records to train an AI model for predicting heart disease risk. By removing identifying information, the organization complies with privacy regulations while benefiting from data-driven insights.

Privacy concern	AI solution	Outcome
Identifiable patient data	Deidentification techniques	Comply with privacy regulations, protect patient confidentiality
Data security	Encryption and access control	Prevent unauthorized access, enhance data security

Mitigating Bias in AI Algorithms

Bias in AI algorithms is a critical ethical issue, as it can lead to unfair or inaccurate healthcare decisions. AI models trained on nonrepresentative or biased data sets may reflect or amplify existing disparities, potentially resulting in unequal treatment for specific population groups.

- *Identifying and addressing bias*: Techniques, such as reweighting data sets, using diverse training data, and performing bias audits help identify and mitigate biases in AI algorithms.
- *Example application:* An AI model used in skin cancer detection is retrained with a diverse data set that includes images of skin tones from various ethnicities, improving its accuracy across different populations.
- *Case scenario*: A hospital implements an AI model to predict patient outcomes in critical care. Initially, the model showed lower accuracy for minority patients. By adding more representative data and conducting regular bias audits, the hospital reduces disparities in the model's predictions.

Type of bias	Mitigation technique	Outcome
Racial bias	Diverse, balanced data sets	Improved accuracy across demographics
Gender bias	Bias auditing and reweighting	Fairer treatment, reduced disparities

Ethical Considerations in AI Deployment

The ethical deployment of AI in healthcare involves ensuring transparency, fairness, and accountability. Ethical concerns include informed consent, maintaining patient autonomy, and ensuring that AI complements human decision-making rather than replacing it.

- *Informed consent and transparency*: Patients should be informed about how AI-driven systems affect their healthcare. Ensuring that patients understand AI's role in their care is essential for preserving trust and autonomy.
- *Example application:* An AI-driven diagnostic tool provides patients with information on how it contributes to their diagnosis, helping them understand the benefits and limitations of AI in their care.
- *Case scenario:* A hospital uses an AI tool to aid in diagnosis but ensures that patients are aware of the tool's involvement and limitations. By doing so, the hospital respects patient autonomy and maintains transparency in care.

Ethical concern	AI-related solution	Outcome
Informed consent	Patient education about AI role	Increased patient trust, maintained autonomy
Decision accountability	Human oversight of AI recommendations	Reduces risk of errors, preserves clinician responsibility

Overview of Regulatory Guidelines and Compliance

Artificial intelligence in healthcare is subject to various regulatory frameworks that ensure patient safety, data security, and ethical usage. Understanding and complying with these regulations is crucial for healthcare organizations deploying AI technologies.

Data Privacy Regulations

Data privacy regulations like HIPAA and GDPR establish guidelines for handling patient data securely and respecting patient privacy rights. Compliance with these regulations is essential for AI applications that use patient information for training or real-time decision-making.

- *HIPAA compliance (US):* The HIPAA privacy rule requires the protection of individually identifiable health information, ensuring that AI applications comply with strict guidelines for data storage, access, and sharing.
- *GDPR compliance (EU):* GDPR mandates robust data protection standards, requiring organizations to obtain explicit patient consent for data usage, enable data portability, and secure data against breaches.

Privacy regulation	Compliance requirement	Impact on AI deployment
HIPAA (US)	Protection of identifiable health data	Limits data sharing, requires deidentification
GDPR (EU)	Explicit consent, data protection	Ensures data security, patient control

Food and Drug Administration and Regulatory Oversight of Artificial Intelligence in Healthcare

In the United States, the Food and Drug Administration (FDA) regulates AI-based medical devices to ensure their safety and efficacy. The FDA's framework includes premarket review, postmarket monitoring, and continuous learning for AI systems that adapt over time.

- *Premarket review:* AI applications classified as medical devices undergo rigorous review before they can be marketed. This process includes evaluating the software's accuracy, clinical validity, and potential risks.
- *Example application:* An AI diagnostic tool for imaging is reviewed by the FDA to ensure it meets safety and efficacy standards before it can be used in hospitals.

FDA requirement	AI system compliance	Outcome
Premarket approval	Thorough testing and validation	Improved safety and reliability in clinical use
Postmarket monitoring	Continuous performance evaluation	Ensures sustained accuracy and effectiveness

Guidelines for Transparency and Explainability

Regulatory bodies emphasize the importance of transparency and explainability in AI systems, ensuring that healthcare providers and patients understand AI-generated recommendations. This transparency helps build trust and enables healthcare providers to make informed decisions.

- *Explainability standards:* AI models used in healthcare should provide explanations for their outputs, especially in high-stakes decisions. Explainable AI techniques help clinicians understand the factors driving AI recommendations.
- *Case scenario:* A hospital adopts an explainable AI tool for stroke prediction. The tool provides a rationale for each prediction, highlighting relevant patient factors. This transparency enables clinicians to trust the tool's output and integrate it into decision-making.

Guideline	AI compliance requirement	Outcome
Explainability	Models must provide transparent reasoning	Increased trust and usability in clinical settings
Transparency in recommendations	AI recommendations accompanied by explanations	Enables informed clinician use and interpretation

Challenges in Implementing Legal, Ethical, and Regulatory Standards

Implementing AI in healthcare comes with challenges related to balancing innovation with legal, ethical, and regulatory compliance. These challenges require continuous monitoring and adaptation as AI technologies evolve.

Balancing Innovation and Compliance

Although regulations aim to protect patients, they may also slow down the adoption of innovative AI technologies. Striking a balance between innovation and compliance requires adaptive regulatory frameworks that accommodate rapid technological advancements.

- *Example challenge:* AI tools that evolve through machine learning require adaptive regulatory approval processes, as their algorithms change over time. Regulatory bodies are exploring frameworks for "adaptive AI" that allow real-time updates without compromising safety.

Challenge	Solution	Outcome
Rapid AI evolution	Adaptive regulatory frameworks	Enables continuous improvement of AI tools
Regulatory delays	Streamlined approval processes	Faster access to beneficial AI technologies

Ensuring Accountability in Artificial Intelligence-driven Healthcare

Accountability in AI-driven healthcare is complex, as responsibility for clinical decisions may be shared between AI systems and human providers. Clear guidelines are needed to assign accountability, ensuring that AI complements human expertise rather than replacing it.

- *Example solution:* Guidelines for shared decision-making, where clinicians retain ultimate accountability for patient care, even when using AI recommendations, help mitigate risks and establish clear lines of responsibility.

Accountability issue	Proposed solution	Outcome
Shared decision-making	Clinician retains final responsibility	Ensures ethical use of AI in clinical settings
AI error handling	Clear protocols for AI error intervention	Reduces risk of harm due to AI misjudgments

Addressing Ethical and Social Implications of Artificial Intelligence in Healthcare

Ethical concerns related to AI in healthcare include the potential loss of human-centered care, as well as social implications, such as unequal access to AI benefits. Addressing these concerns requires a commitment to ethical principles and equitable healthcare delivery.

- *Example solution*: Developing ethical frameworks that prioritize human-centered care and equitable access to AI technologies helps mitigate social and ethical risks.

Ethical concern	Mitigation strategy	Outcome
Loss of human-centered care	Ensure AI complements, not replaces, clinicians	Preserves quality of care and empathy
Unequal access to AI benefits	Implement equitable access policies	Reduces healthcare disparities

FUTURE DIRECTIONS FOR LEGAL, ETHICAL, AND REGULATORY STANDARDS IN AI HEALTHCARE

- *Global harmonization of AI regulations:* Develop international standards to streamline AI deployment across countries, balancing innovation with legal, ethical, and data privacy requirements.
- *Dynamic regulatory frameworks for adaptive AI:* Create frameworks for continuously evolving AI systems, allowing safe and compliant updates to algorithms without disrupting clinical applications.
- *Transparent AI accountability mechanisms:* Establish clear guidelines delineating accountability between clinicians and AI tools, ensuring ethical use while maintaining human oversight.

CONCLUSION

Artificial intelligence in healthcare presents unprecedented opportunities for improving patient care, but it also raises complex legal, ethical, and regulatory challenges. Addressing privacy, bias, accountability, and transparency is essential for deploying AI responsibly and building trust among patients and healthcare providers.

As AI technology advances, adaptive and collaborative regulatory frameworks will be critical to ensuring the safe, ethical, and equitable use of AI in healthcare. The future of AI in healthcare requires a balance between innovation and compliance, guided by principles that prioritize patient welfare, ethical integrity, and regulatory oversight. By addressing these considerations, healthcare systems can harness AI's full potential while maintaining the highest standards of safety and care.

Implementing Artificial Intelligence in Clinical Practice

INTRODUCTION

Artificial intelligence (AI) has the potential to revolutionize clinical practice by enhancing diagnostic accuracy, treatment planning, patient monitoring, and healthcare outcomes. However, integrating AI into clinical workflows presents challenges that span technological, organizational, and human factors. Successfully implementing AI in healthcare settings requires strategic planning, addressing interoperability, ensuring clinician buy-in, and fostering collaboration between AI developers and healthcare providers. This chapter explores the key challenges and solutions for integrating AI into diverse healthcare environments, along with best practices for building successful partnerships between AI developers and clinicians.

Challenges and Solutions for Integrating Artificial Intelligence in Diverse Healthcare Settings

Implementing AI in clinical practice involves overcoming technical, operational, and cultural barriers. Addressing these challenges ensures that AI systems are effectively integrated into workflows and deliver real benefits to healthcare providers and patients.

Data Quality and Interoperability Challenges

Artificial intelligence systems rely on high-quality, standardized data for training and operational use. However, healthcare data often exist in disparate formats and systems, making it challenging to achieve interoperability and data consistency across diverse healthcare settings.

- *Data integration and standardization:* AI integration requires data from various sources, including electronic health records, imaging systems, and laboratory data. Ensuring consistent data formats and adopting interoperability standards like Fast Healthcare Interoperability Resources (FHIR) facilitates data sharing between the systems.
- *Solution:* Implement data integration platforms that harmonize data from different systems, enabling AI algorithms to access comprehensive, high-quality data sets for analysis.
- *Case scenario:* A hospital implements an AI-driven predictive analytics tool for sepsis detection. Initially, the data formats across different departments are incompatible. By adopting interoperability standards and using data integration tools, the hospital successfully integrates the AI system into its electronic health record, allowing seamless data flow and real-time predictions.

Challenge	Solution	Outcome
Data inconsistency across systems	Data integration and standardization	Improved data quality, reliable AI predictions
Lack of interoperability	Adoption of FHIR and other standards	Seamless integration with existing systems

Workflow Integration and Usability

Integrating AI into clinical workflows requires thoughtful consideration of how clinicians interact with AI tools. AI systems that disrupt established workflows or are difficult to use may be met with resistance, limiting their impact on clinical practice.

- *Solution*: Conduct workflow analysis to ensure that AI tools align with clinicians' existing practices. Involve healthcare providers in the design and testing phases to enhance usability and ensure that AI tools support, rather than disrupt, clinical workflows.
- *Case scenario:* An AI diagnostic tool for radiology is introduced at a hospital, but radiologists find that its interface is unintuitive, slowing down their workflow. The developers work with radiologists to redesign the interface, making it more user-friendly and enabling faster image analysis, which improves adoption.

Challenge	Solution	Outcome
Poor workflow fit	Workflow analysis and clinician involvement	Enhanced usability, improved adoption
Complex user interfaces	Simplified and intuitive design	Increased user satisfaction, efficient workflow

Clinician Trust and Acceptance

Clinician acceptance is critical for successful AI implementation. Factors affecting trust include AI accuracy, transparency, and alignment with clinical judgment. Ensuring that clinicians understand AI's role in augmenting—rather than replacing—their expertise is key to fostering trust.

- *Solution*: Build trust by implementing explainable AI (XAI) that provides transparency into how AI models make decisions. Provide training sessions to familiarize clinicians with AI capabilities and limitations and promote a collaborative approach to AI usage.
- *Case scenario:* A hospital introduces an AI tool for predicting readmission risk, but clinicians are initially hesitant to trust its recommendations. The developers add explainability features, allowing clinicians to view the factors driving each prediction. Regular workshops are also conducted, leading to greater acceptance and integration of the tool into patient discharge planning.

Challenge	Solution	Outcome
Clinician skepticism	Use of XAI and training	Increased trust and usage of AI in decision-making
Fear of replacement	Education on AI's supportive role	Improved clinician acceptance and engagement

Data Privacy and Security Concerns

Artificial intelligence systems often require access to sensitive patient data, raising concerns about data privacy and security. Ensuring compliance with regulations, such as Health Insurance Portability and Accountability Act of 1996 (HIPAA) and General Data Protection Regulation (GDPR) is essential to protect patient information and maintain public trust.

- *Solution:* Implement robust data encryption, secure access controls, and anonymization techniques. Regularly audit AI systems to ensure they comply with data privacy regulations and engage in transparent communication about data usage.
- *Case scenario:* An AI-powered telemedicine platform uses patient data for predictive analytics. To ensure data privacy, the platform employs advanced encryption and restricts access to authorized personnel only. These measures help the platform comply with HIPAA, building patient trust in the technology.

Challenge	Solution	Outcome
Data security risks	Encryption and secure access controls	Enhanced data protection, regulatory compliance
Privacy concerns	Data anonymization and transparency	Increased patient and provider trust

Financial and Resource Constraints

The implementation of AI systems requires significant financial investment and technical resources, which can be challenging for healthcare organizations with limited budgets.

- *Solution*: Start with pilot programs or scalable AI projects to assess return on investment (ROI) before larger investments. Seek partnerships or grants to support funding and consider using open-source AI tools to reduce costs.
- *Case scenario:* A small clinic wants to adopt AI for patient triage but faces budget constraints. By collaborating with a local university, the clinic secures funding for a pilot program. Positive results from the pilot justify further investment in AI, enabling the clinic to implement the technology more widely.

Challenge	Solution	Outcome
Budget limitations	Pilot programs and partnerships	Cost-effective AI implementation
Resource scarcity	Use of open-source and scalable solutions	Reduced financial burden, accessibility to AI benefits

Best Practices for Collaboration Between Artificial Intelligence Developers and Healthcare Providers

Successful AI integration requires collaboration between AI developers and healthcare providers to ensure that solutions meet clinical needs and align with healthcare workflows. Best practices include regular communication, joint problem-solving, and continuous feedback.

Involve Clinicians in the Development Process

Involving clinicians in the AI development process ensures that solutions address real clinical needs and are usable in healthcare settings. Clinicians provide insights into workflow requirements, patient needs, and the specific challenges they face.

- *Practice:* Include clinicians in each phase of AI development—from design to testing—and gather their feedback to refine the product. Regular meetings help ensure alignment between technical and clinical perspectives.
- *Case scenario:* An AI developer team working on a diagnostic tool collaborates with clinicians throughout development. Clinician input helps fine-tune the tool's user interface and ensure that its recommendations align with clinical guidelines, leading to a more effective final product.

Practice	Benefits	Outcome
Clinician involvement in design	Ensures alignment with clinical needs	Improved relevance and usability of AI tools
Regular feedback sessions	Continuous product improvement	Enhanced functionality and user satisfaction

Establish Clear Communication Channels

Effective communication between AI developers and healthcare providers is essential for managing expectations, addressing challenges, and fostering collaboration. Clear communication channels facilitate knowledge exchange and ensure that all stakeholders understand project goals.

- *Practice:* Set up regular meetings, collaborative platforms, and clear points of contact for both teams. Document and share progress updates, technical adjustments, and any issues encountered to keep everyone informed.
- *Case scenario:* A healthcare organization implementing an AI system for patient scheduling holds weekly check-ins with the development team. These meetings provide a forum for discussing challenges, such as technical integration issues, and identifying solutions quickly.

Practice	Benefits	Outcome
Regular meetings and updates	Keep all parties informed	Faster problem-solving, smoother implementation
Collaborative platforms	Facilitate knowledge sharing	Stronger alignment and better communication

Educate Clinicians on AI Capabilities and Limitations

Providing clinicians with training on AI tools' capabilities and limitations helps manage expectations and ensure responsible usage. Clinicians need to understand when and how to rely on AI outputs and be aware of their limitations in specific contexts.

- *Practice:* Conduct training sessions and provide educational resources on AI basics, model interpretation, and ethical considerations. Encourage clinicians to question AI outputs and use their judgment to make final decisions.
- *Case scenario:* A hospital introduces an AI tool for triaging emergency cases. Training sessions are held to explain the tool's predictive capabilities and limitations, helping clinicians understand when to trust its recommendations and when to rely on their clinical judgment.

Practice	Benefits	Outcome
AI education and training	Informed and responsible AI usage	Increased clinician confidence and improved patient care
Emphasis on clinical judgment	Ensures AI augments rather than replaces judgment	Balanced AI integration in clinical practice

Implement Continuous Evaluation and Feedback Loops

Continuous evaluation of AI systems ensures that they meet clinical goals and maintain accuracy over time. Feedback loops allow healthcare providers to share insights from real-world use, enabling developers to refine AI tools based on practical experiences.

- *Practice:* Establish feedback loops with clinicians, where they can report issues, suggest improvements, and track AI performance. Regular updates based on feedback ensure that the AI system evolves to meet clinical needs.
- *Case scenario:* A predictive model for intensive care unit (ICU) admissions is implemented in a hospital. Clinicians provide regular feedback on its accuracy, leading the development team to adjust the model parameters for improved predictions, resulting in better patient care.

Practice	Benefits	Outcome
Continuous feedback from clinicians	Ongoing product refinement	Higher accuracy and relevance in clinical use
Performance monitoring	Ensures model reliability over time	Sustained quality and efficacy of AI system

Future Directions for Implementing Artificial Intelligence in Clinical Practice

- *Hybrid human-AI clinical decision models:* Develop integrated frameworks where AI supports but does not replace clinician judgment, combining computational precision with human expertise for nuanced decisions.
- *Scalable AI solutions for resource-limited settings:* Create cost-effective AI systems that operate with minimal computational resources, making advanced technologies accessible to rural and underfunded healthcare facilities.
- *Continuous AI feedback systems in clinical settings:* Implement feedback loops between clinicians and developers to refine AI tools based on real-world usage, ensuring alignment with clinical needs and improving outcomes.

CONCLUSION

Implementing AI in clinical practice requires overcoming various challenges related to data interoperability, workflow integration, clinician acceptance, and data privacy. Solutions, such as standardizing data, ensuring usability, fostering clinician trust, and providing education are crucial for effective integration. Additionally, collaboration between AI developers and healthcare providers is essential for developing AI tools that address real clinical needs and fit seamlessly into healthcare workflows.

As AI technology continues to evolve, the future of AI in clinical practice will involve adaptive models, hybrid decision-making frameworks, and expanded training for clinicians. By adhering to best practices and fostering collaboration, healthcare systems can harness the full potential of AI to improve patient outcomes, streamline operations, and enhance the quality of care.

21

Future Directions and Innovations in Artificial Intelligence for Medicine

INTRODUCTION

Artificial intelligence (AI) is rapidly advancing across various fields, with significant impacts on healthcare. From diagnostic imaging to personalized medicine, AI-driven innovations are reshaping how healthcare is delivered, increasing precision, efficiency, and accessibility. As AI continues to evolve, new trends and advancements are expected to emerge, offering even greater potential for transforming patient care. However, realizing this potential requires preparation, continuous education, and adaptation among healthcare professionals. This chapter explores emerging trends and future innovations in AI for healthcare, along with strategies for physicians to stay updated and engaged with AI advancements.

Emerging Trends and Advancements in Artificial Intelligence for Healthcare

The field of AI in healthcare is dynamic, with new developments regularly enhancing how healthcare providers diagnose, treat, and manage patient care. Key emerging trends include the expansion of AI in predictive analytics, personalized medicine, drug discovery, and digital health.

Expansion of Predictive Analytics for Proactive Healthcare

Predictive analytics in healthcare uses historical data, machine learning models, and real-time patient information to predict health risks and outcomes. This trend is moving toward proactive, preventative care, enabling clinicians to address potential health issues before they become critical.

- *AI for early disease detection:* Advanced algorithms analyze risk factors and genetic information to identify individuals at high risk for diseases, such as cancer, cardiovascular disease, and diabetes.
- *Example application*: AI algorithms are applied to electronic health record data to identify patients at high risk of developing heart disease. This allows healthcare providers to implement early interventions, potentially preventing heart disease or reducing its severity.
- *Case scenario*: A healthcare provider uses an AI tool to analyze a patient population's electronic health record data. The tool identifies individuals at high risk for stroke, prompting the provider to implement preventive measures, such as lifestyle changes and medication adjustments.

Health condition	AI predictive role	Outcome
Cardiovascular disease	Identifies high-risk individuals	Preventive interventions, reduced incidence
Diabetes	Predicts risk based on lifestyle/genetic factors	Early management, better long-term outcomes

Advancements in Personalized Medicine

Personalized medicine tailors treatments to individual patients based on genetic, lifestyle, and environmental factors. AI plays a critical role in analyzing complex datasets to provide personalized recommendations for medication, treatment plans, and preventive care.

- *Precision drug therapy and pharmacogenomics*: AI-driven analysis of genetic data enables clinicians to prescribe medications based on a patient's genetic profile, enhancing drug efficacy and reducing adverse reactions.
- *Example application:* AI algorithms analyze genomic data to predict which patients will respond best to specific cancer treatments, enabling oncologists to customize therapy plans and optimize treatment outcomes.
- *Case scenario*: An oncologist uses an AI tool to analyze a patient's genetic profile, identifying a targeted therapy with the highest likelihood of effectiveness. This approach reduces the need for trial-and-error treatment and improves the patient's prognosis.

Treatment type	AI's role in personalization	Outcome
Cancer therapy	Analyzes genetic data for drug response	Tailored treatment, improved efficacy
Antidepressant medication	Predicts response based on genetic profile	Reduced side effects, better mental health outcomes

AI-Driven Drug Discovery and Development

Artificial intelligence is accelerating drug discovery and development by analyzing vast datasets, predicting molecular interactions, and identifying potential drug candidates. This reduces the time and cost of drug development, bringing effective treatments to market faster.

- *AI for target identification and lead optimization*: AI algorithms predict how different molecules interact with biological targets, helping pharmaceutical companies identify promising drug candidates and refine them for better efficacy.
- *Example application*: Deep learning models analyze protein structures to discover molecules that could inhibit viral replication, such as for COVID-19 treatments.
- *Case scenario*: A pharmaceutical company uses an AI model to screen millions of compounds, identifying a handful of candidates that could potentially treat Alzheimer's disease. This accelerates the early stages of drug discovery and helps prioritize compounds for further testing.

Phase of drug development	AI contribution	Outcome
Target identification	Predicts potential biological targets	Faster discovery of promising drug targets
Lead optimization	Analyzes molecular interactions	Improved drug efficacy, reduced side effects

Expansion of Digital Health and Remote Monitoring

Digital health technologies and AI-enabled remote monitoring support continuous patient observation, enabling early detection of complications and improving chronic disease management. This trend is particularly valuable in managing patients with limited access to in-person care.

- *Wearable devices and Internet of Things (IoT) integration:* Wearable devices collect real-time health data, which AI models analyze to detect anomalies, such as irregular heart rhythms, early signs of infection, or fluctuations in glucose levels.

- *Example application:* AI-driven apps integrate with wearables to monitor heart rates and detect irregularities, alerting users to seek medical attention if needed.
- *Case scenario*: A patient with heart disease uses a wearable device linked to an AI-powered app. The app continuously monitors the patient's heart rate, detecting an irregular pattern and sending an alert. The patient visits their doctor, who diagnoses arrhythmia and adjusts their treatment plan.

Health monitoring	AI's role in analysis	Outcome
Heart rhythm monitoring	Detects arrhythmias in real time	Early detection, timely intervention
Glucose monitoring for diabetes	Tracks glucose patterns and alerts anomalies	Improved blood sugar management, reduced complications

AI in Robotic-assisted Surgery and Real-time Decision Support

Artificial intelligence applications in robotic-assisted surgery enhance precision and accuracy, allowing for minimally invasive procedures. Additionally, real-time AI-based decision support systems provide insights and recommendations to assist surgeons and clinicians during procedures.

- *Example application:* AI-powered robotic systems guide surgeons in complex procedures, reducing variability and enhancing precision in surgeries like prostatectomy and cardiac surgery.
- *Case scenario*: A surgeon uses a robotic-assisted system with AI guidance for a delicate spinal procedure. AI provides real-time feedback on anatomical structures, helping the surgeon avoid nerves and ensuring precise implant placement.

Surgical application	AI's role in support	Outcome
Robotic spinal surgery	Real-time anatomical guidance	Increased precision, reduced complication risk
Cardiac surgery	Minimally invasive AI-assisted interventions	Shorter recovery times, improved patient outcomes

Preparing for Future Developments and Continuous Education in Artificial Intelligence for Physicians

As AI technology in healthcare continues to evolve, it is essential for healthcare professionals to stay informed, develop new skills, and adapt to emerging AI tools. Continuous education and training are critical for physicians to maximize the benefits of AI in their practice.

Incorporating AI Education Into Medical Training

Medical schools and residency programs are beginning to incorporate AI and data science education into their curricula, preparing future physicians to understand and leverage AI in clinical settings.

- *Example application:* Medical schools offer courses on AI fundamentals, machine learning, and data interpretation, ensuring that new physicians understand how to use AI tools ethically and effectively.
- *Case scenario*: A medical school integrates an AI module into its curriculum, covering the basics of machine learning and its applications in medicine. Students learn how to interpret AI-generated predictions and integrate them into clinical decision-making.

Education level	AI curriculum focus	Outcome
Medical school	Introduction to AI and data science	Future-ready physicians with AI literacy
Residency	Applied AI for clinical specialties	Skill development in AI-supported patient care

Continuous Professional Development in AI for Practicing Physicians

Continuous education programs, workshops, and certifications on AI applications in healthcare allow practicing physicians to stay current with AI advancements and integrate new tools into their clinical practice.

- *Example application*: Healthcare institutions offer AI-focused workshops and online courses on topics such as predictive analytics, robotic surgery, and personalized medicine, equipping physicians with practical AI skills.
- *Case scenario*: A healthcare provider offers an AI workshop for its staff, covering predictive analytics and its applications in patient risk assessment. The training enables physicians to integrate predictive models into their workflows, enhancing patient care.

Professional development format	Focus area	Outcome
Workshops and seminars	Practical AI skills in clinical settings	Improved physician confidence in using AI
Online certification programs	Advanced AI applications	Credentialed expertise, enhanced patient outcomes

Developing Collaborative Skills for AI-Healthcare Teams

Collaboration between healthcare professionals and AI developers is essential for creating effective AI tools. Physicians with knowledge of AI can contribute to the development process, ensuring tools meet clinical needs and align with healthcare workflows.

- *Example application:* Collaborative programs bring together clinicians, data scientists, and developers, allowing them to codesign AI applications tailored to specific medical needs.
- *Case scenario*: A hospital creates an interdisciplinary team to develop an AI tool for early sepsis detection. Physicians provide insights into clinical workflows and data requirements, whereas developers ensure the tool integrates smoothly into the hospital's system.

Collaboration type	Focus	Outcome
Interdisciplinary AI-healthcare teams	Codesign of clinically relevant AI tools	Enhanced tool usability, improved healthcare outcomes
Clinician input in development	Workflow alignment and relevance	Higher adoption and effectiveness of AI

Staying Informed of AI Regulatory and Ethical Standards

As AI technologies evolve, new ethical and regulatory standards are introduced. Physicians must stay updated on these standards to ensure that AI tools are used responsibly and in compliance with legal requirements.

- *Example application*: Continuous education programs offer updates on regulatory frameworks and ethical guidelines, equipping physicians to evaluate AI tools critically.
- *Case scenario*: A physician attends a workshop on ethical AI use in healthcare, learning about privacy considerations, bias mitigation, and patient consent in AI applications. This knowledge helps them make informed decisions about implementing AI in patient care.

Focus area	Educational content	Outcome
Regulatory updates	Understanding compliance requirements	Legal and ethical AI usage in clinical practice
Ethical considerations	Addressing bias, privacy, and consent	Improved patient trust, ethical AI implementation

Future Directions for AI-Driven Healthcare Innovation

- *AI-powered precision public health:* Expand AI to analyze multiomics data (genomics, proteomics) for predicting disease trends at the population level, enabling tailored public health initiatives.
- *Federated learning for collaborative AI development:* Promote federated learning to enable AI models to learn from diverse datasets across institutions while preserving patient privacy, enhancing model generalizability.
- *AI integration in home-based care models:* Advance AI-enabled home monitoring systems for chronic disease management, reducing hospital visits and improving patient autonomy through proactive care.

CONCLUSION

Artificial intelligence in healthcare is advancing rapidly, with transformative potential across various medical applications. Emerging trends in predictive analytics, personalized medicine, digital health, and robotic-assisted surgery are paving the way for more efficient and precise patient care. However, to realize the full potential of AI in clinical practice, continuous education, interdisciplinary collaboration, and a commitment to ethical standards are essential.

As the field progresses, healthcare providers who stay informed about AI developments and actively engage with new technologies will be well-positioned to improve patient outcomes and drive innovation in healthcare. The future of AI in medicine holds immense promise, but achieving its full impact requires a proactive, educated, and collaborative healthcare community dedicated to embracing the future of intelligent healthcare delivery.

22 Case Studies and Real-World Applications of Artificial Intelligence in Healthcare

INTRODUCTION

The impact of artificial intelligence (AI) in healthcare is best illustrated through real-world case studies that demonstrate how AI-driven technologies are enhancing clinical outcomes across various medical specialties. From radiology and oncology to cardiology and primary care, AI applications have transformed diagnostics, treatment planning, patient management, and healthcare delivery. This chapter presents detailed case studies from different clinical domains, highlighting the benefits, challenges, and lessons learned from integrating AI into clinical practice.

Case Study 1: Artificial Intelligence in Radiology—Enhancing Diagnostic Accuracy

Radiology is one of the earliest and most successful fields in adopting AI for clinical use, primarily due to the abundance of imaging data and the high demand for accurate diagnostics.

Overview and Implementation

An AI-based image recognition tool was integrated into the radiology department of a major hospital to assist radiologists in detecting lung nodules on chest X-rays and computed tomography (CT) scans. This tool used deep learning algorithms trained on millions of radiographic images, allowing it to identify potential nodules with high accuracy.

- *Artificial intelligence tool function*: The tool analyzed images and highlighted suspicious areas for review, offering a "second opinion" to radiologists, particularly for detecting early-stage lung cancer.
- *Case scenario:* During routine lung cancer screenings, the AI tool flagged a subtle nodule in a patient's chest X-ray that was initially missed by the radiologist. Further investigation confirmed an early-stage lung cancer diagnosis, enabling early intervention and improving the patient's prognosis.

Impact	Outcome
Improved nodule detection	Increased detection rate for early-stage lung cancer
Reduced missed diagnoses	Enhanced radiologist accuracy and confidence

Lessons Learned

- *Enhancing accuracy with human–AI collaboration:* The AI tool's ability to flag subtle findings improved diagnostic accuracy, but human oversight was crucial for confirming results.

- *Building trust with transparency*: Radiologists were more likely to trust the AI tool after seeing transparent explanations of its detections.

Case Study 2: Artificial Intelligence in Oncology—Personalized Treatment Planning

Artificial intelligence's role in oncology is expanding, particularly in creating personalized treatment plans based on genomic, clinical, and imaging data.

Overview and Implementation

An AI-based precision medicine platform was implemented in an oncology clinic to aid oncologists in creating personalized treatment regimens for patients with breast cancer. This platform analyzed patients' genetic profiles, tumor characteristics, and treatment history to recommend tailored therapies.

- *AI tool function*: The tool provided oncologists with insights into the most effective treatment options based on individual patient data and the latest clinical research.
- *Case scenario:* A patient diagnosed with an aggressive form of breast cancer received a treatment recommendation from the AI platform, which suggested a combination therapy tailored to her genetic profile. This personalized approach improved her response to treatment, reducing tumor size more effectively than standard therapies.

Impact	Outcome
Enhanced treatment personalization	Higher treatment efficacy and reduced side effects
Reduced trial and error	Faster optimization of effective therapy

Lessons Learned

- *Interdisciplinary collaboration*: Integrating AI requires close collaboration between oncologists, geneticists, and AI developers.
- *Continuous learning and updates*: Regular updates to the AI system ensured that recommendations remained aligned with the latest oncology research.

Case Study 3: Artificial Intelligence in Cardiology—Predictive Analytics for Heart Failure Management

Artificial intelligence-driven predictive analytics has become instrumental in managing chronic diseases, such as heart failure, by identifying patients at risk and enabling preventive measures.

Overview and Implementation

A predictive analytics tool was implemented in a cardiology department to forecast heart failure exacerbations in patients with chronic heart disease. The tool analyzed patients' clinical data, lifestyle factors, and medication adherence to predict the likelihood of an acute episode.

- *AI tool function:* The system generated risk scores for each patient, allowing cardiologists to prioritize high-risk patients for follow-up and intervention.
- *Case scenario:* A patient with chronic heart failure had an elevated risk score from the AI tool, indicating a likely exacerbation within the next month. The cardiology team adjusted

the patient's medication and scheduled closer monitoring, successfully preventing hospitalization.

Impact	Outcome
Early risk identification	Reduced emergency admissions
Proactive management	Improved patient stability and quality of life

Lessons Learned

- *Empowering preventive care*: The predictive tool enabled proactive interventions that improved patient outcomes and reduced hospital costs.
- *Importance of data quality*: Reliable predictions depend on high-quality, comprehensive patient data, emphasizing the need for accurate and complete electronic health record documentation.

Case Study 4: Artificial Intelligence in Emergency Medicine—Triage and Decision Support

In emergency medicine, AI assists in patient triage, improving response times and outcomes for critical conditions, such as sepsis and stroke.

Overview and Implementation

An AI-driven triage system was deployed in the emergency department (ED) of a busy urban hospital to prioritize patients presenting with symptoms of sepsis. The tool analyzed vital signs and lab results in real time, identifying patients at risk and alerting healthcare staff.

- *AI tool function:* The triage system calculated a sepsis risk score based on real-time data, helping ED staff quickly identify high-risk patients.
- *Case scenario:* A patient arrived at the ED with mild symptoms. The AI tool flagged a high sepsis risk based on abnormal lab values and vital signs, prompting immediate intervention. Rapid treatment prevented sepsis progression, reducing the patient's length of stay and potential complications.

Impact	Outcome
Rapid sepsis identification	Faster treatment initiation, reduced mortality
Improved triage efficiency	Enhanced ED workflow and patient outcomes

Lessons Learned

- *Importance of real-time data*: The success of the AI tool relied on real-time data integration to provide accurate, actionable alerts.
- *Team training:* Training ED staff to interpret and act on AI alerts was essential for rapid response and effective use of the system.

Case Study 5: Artificial Intelligence in Primary Care—Virtual Health Assistants for Patient Engagement

Virtual health assistants powered by AI support primary care by improving patient engagement, adherence, and health literacy through personalized education and reminders.

Overview and Implementation

A primary care clinic introduced a virtual health assistant to engage patients with chronic conditions, including diabetes and hypertension. The assistant provided educational resources, medication reminders, and lifestyle tips tailored to each patient's health profile.

- *AI tool function*: The virtual assistant used natural language processing to interact with patients, answer questions, and provide personalized health advice.
- *Case scenario:* A patient with hypertension and diabetes used the virtual health assistant to track her medication and receive daily reminders. The assistant also provided dietary tips and answered questions about her condition, leading to better adherence and improved blood pressure control.

Impact	Outcome
Improved patient adherence	Enhanced medication compliance, better disease control
Increased health literacy	Empowered patients with knowledge of self-care

Lessons Learned

- *Patient-centric design*: Personalizing interactions based on individual patient needs increased engagement and effectiveness.
- *Empowering self-management:* The virtual assistant facilitated self-management, which is crucial for managing chronic conditions in primary care settings.

Case Study 6: Artificial Intelligence in Surgery—Robotic-Assisted Surgery for Enhanced Precision

Artificial intelligence-driven robotic systems are being used to assist surgeons in performing minimally invasive procedures with high precision, improving patient outcomes and reducing recovery times.

Overview and Implementation

A robotic-assisted surgical system was introduced in a hospital's urology department to aid in prostate surgeries. The AI-driven robot provided real-time guidance and enhanced visualization and stability, helping surgeons make precise incisions and reduce tissue damage.

- *AI tool function:* The system offered real-time feedback on anatomical structures, enabling the surgeon to maintain precision and avoid critical areas during surgery.
- *Case scenario:* A patient underwent a robotic-assisted prostatectomy. The AI system's real-time guidance helped the surgeon avoid nerve bundles, reducing the risk of postoperative complications and leading to quicker recovery.

Impact	Outcome
Enhanced surgical precision	Reduced complications, faster recovery
Minimally invasive approach	Decreased hospital stay, improved patient satisfaction

Lessons Learned

- *Augmenting surgeon skills with AI:* The robotic system enhanced surgical precision, but surgeon expertise remained essential for decision-making.

- *Investment in training:* Surgeons required specialized training to operate AI-driven robotic systems effectively, highlighting the need for continued education.

Lessons Learned and Insights From Clinical Integration of AI

The successful implementation of AI in healthcare depends on various factors, including data quality, collaboration, and clinician education. The following insights summarize key lessons from these case studies:

- *Human–AI collaboration:* AI is most effective when it complements, rather than replaces, human expertise. The best outcomes were achieved when clinicians used AI as a support tool while retaining oversight.
- *Importance of data quality and integration:* High-quality, interoperable data are essential for AI models to function effectively. Data standardization and real-time integration were recurring challenges but critical for success.
- *Transparency and explainability:* Clinicians are more likely to trust AI tools that provide clear, explainable results. Explainable AI builds confidence and ensures clinicians understand the rationale behind AI recommendations.
- *Ongoing education and training:* Continuous education for clinicians and healthcare staff on AI's capabilities, limitations, and ethical considerations is vital for successful adoption. Training helps users leverage AI tools effectively and maintain patient safety.
- *Patient-centric approaches:* AI applications that prioritize patient engagement and empowerment, such as virtual health assistants, show significant promise in enhancing patient adherence and satisfaction, particularly in chronic disease management.
- *Continuous monitoring and evaluation:* Regular performance monitoring and feedback loops are essential to ensure AI tools maintain their accuracy and relevance over time, allowing adjustments to align with evolving clinical needs and advancements in medical knowledge.

CONCLUSION

Real-world case studies illustrate the transformative potential of AI in healthcare, enhancing diagnostics, personalized treatment, predictive analytics, and patient engagement across specialties. Although the benefits are clear, the successful integration of AI requires a thoughtful approach, emphasizing collaboration between AI developers and healthcare providers, continuous education, and adherence to ethical standards.

As AI continues to evolve, these lessons and insights will guide future implementations, enabling healthcare systems to maximize the potential of AI while prioritizing patient safety and quality of care. The journey of AI in healthcare is ongoing, and learning from these real-world applications will pave the way for further innovations that support clinicians and improve patient outcomes.

Self-assessment—
Multiple-Choice Questions (MCQs)

1. Which of the following is a primary challenge in implementing artificial intelligence (AI) in clinical practice?
   A. Lack of accurate data integration
   B. High patient acceptance
   C. Simplified workflow integration
   D. Lack of regulatory oversight

   Answer: A. Lack of accurate data integration

   Explanation: AI applications in clinical practice often struggle with integrating data from multiple sources due to variability in data standards and formats across healthcare systems. Accurate data integration is essential for AI tools to function correctly, as poor data quality can reduce model reliability and effectiveness.

2. In AI-assisted radiology, how does deep learning improve diagnostic accuracy for conditions, such as lung nodules?
   A. By automating all imaging analysis without human oversight
   B. Through analyzing genetic data instead of imaging data
   C. By identifying subtle patterns that might be overlooked by human radiologists
   D. By reducing the need for any clinician interaction

   Answer: C. By identifying subtle patterns that might be overlooked by human radiologists

   Explanation: Deep learning algorithms in radiology can detect subtle patterns in imaging data, such as small or ambiguous lung nodules, that might be missed by human eyes, enhancing diagnostic sensitivity and supporting early disease detection.

3. What is a significant benefit of AI in personalized medicine, particularly in oncology?
   A. It replaces the need for traditional chemotherapy
   B. It provides a generalized treatment for all cancer patients
   C. It allows tailoring treatments to individual genetic profiles
   D. It decreases the need for patient data in treatment planning

   Answer: C. It allows tailoring treatments to individual genetic profiles

   Explanation: AI enables personalized treatment plans in oncology by analyzing a patient's genetic information, which can identify mutations or biomarkers that make them more likely to respond to specific therapies, resulting in improved outcomes.

4. Which ethical concern is central to deploying AI in clinical practice, particularly in predictive analytics?
   A. Overestimating AI's capabilities
   B. Transparency of decision-making processes
   C. Lack of data anonymization
   D. Over-reliance on human intervention

   Answer: B. Transparency of decision-making processes
   Explanation: In predictive analytics, it is essential to maintain transparency in how AI models reach conclusions. Explainable AI methods can help clinicians understand and trust AI recommendations, ensuring that the decision-making process is clear and ethical.

5. How does federated learning contribute to AI's role in healthcare?
   A. By aggregating patient data in one centralized server
   B. By training models without sharing sensitive patient data across institutions
   C. By increasing patient participation in data collection
   D. By providing real-time feedback to patients

   Answer: B. By training models without sharing sensitive patient data across institutions
   Explanation: Federated learning allows AI models to train on data from multiple institutions without transferring sensitive patient information to a central server, protecting patient privacy while enabling comprehensive model training.

6. In AI-driven diagnostic tools for cardiology, which aspect improves heart failure management?
   A. Prediction of likely disease progression based on past data
   B. Elimination of all manual diagnostic processes
   C. Restricting data usage to demographic data only
   D. Generalizing treatment plans across populations

   Answer: A. Prediction of likely disease progression based on past data
   Explanation: Predictive analytics in cardiology uses historical data to forecast disease progression, allowing early intervention and personalized management strategies, particularly for chronic conditions, such as heart failure.

7. What role does data deidentification play in AI's ethical deployment in healthcare?
   A. It personalizes patient recommendations
   B. It enables the use of patient-specific data without privacy risks
   C. It allows unrestricted sharing of patient information
   D. It eliminates the need for data security protocols

   Answer: B. It enables the use of patient-specific data without privacy risks
   Explanation: Deidentification processes remove identifiable information from datasets, allowing AI models to analyze patient data for insights while maintaining privacy and complying with regulations, such as Health Insurance Portability and Accountability Act of 1996 (HIPAA) and General Data Protection Regulation (GDPR).

8. Which AI model type is most commonly used in detecting anomalies in radiology images?
   A. Decision trees
   B. Support vector machines
   C. Convolutional neural networks (CNNs)
   D. K-nearest neighbors

Answer: C. Convolutional neural networks (CNNs)

Explanation: CNNs are widely used in medical imaging due to their ability to process and interpret visual data, making them ideal for identifying patterns in radiology images, such as tumors or fractures.

9. How does AI improve adherence to medication among patients with chronic diseases?
   A. By replacing human intervention in therapy
   B. Through personalized reminders and behavioral nudges
   C. By standardizing medication schedules across all patients
   D. By decreasing the frequency of patient follow-ups

   Answer: B. Through personalized reminders and behavioral nudges

   Explanation: AI-powered systems send reminders and nudges based on patient behavior patterns, helping improve adherence to medication schedules, especially for patients managing chronic conditions.

10. In the context of AI-powered virtual assistants, which functionality directly supports patient empowerment?
    A. Limiting patient access to health information
    B. Providing tailored education and real-time responses to patient inquiries
    C. Replacing primary care visits with automated diagnosis
    D. Restricting patient interaction to emergency scenarios only

    Answer: B. Providing tailored education and real-time responses to patient inquiries

    Explanation: Virtual health assistants educate patients about their conditions and answer questions, which empowers them with the knowledge needed to participate actively in their care and make informed decisions.

11. *Case:* A 55-year-old male with a history of hypertension and obesity visits his cardiologist. The clinic recently implemented an AI-powered predictive tool that analyzes patient data to assess the risk of myocardial infarction (MI) within the next 5 years. Based on the AI-generated risk score, the cardiologist suggests lifestyle modifications and starts the patient on statin therapy.

    Question: What AI capability is primarily responsible for this risk assessment?
    A. Natural language processing (NLP)
    B. Predictive analytics using machine learning algorithms
    C. Robotic process automation (RPA)
    D. Federated learning

    Answer: B. Predictive analytics using machine learning algorithms

    Explanation: Predictive analytics uses historical data, such as risk factors and demographic information, to generate risk scores for conditions like MI. Machine learning algorithms analyze these data points, enabling clinicians to make proactive management decisions for high-risk patients.

12. *Case:* A hospital uses an AI-based early warning system (EWS) that continuously monitors intensive care unit (ICU) patients' vital signs. The system flags a patient's vitals as abnormal and predicts a high likelihood of septic shock within the next hour, alerting the medical team to initiate early interventions.

Question: What is the key factor in the effectiveness of this AI-based early warning system?

A. High patient-to-nurse ratio
B. Real-time data processing and continuous monitoring
C. Limiting access to only senior physicians
D. Replacing human intervention entirely

Answer: B. Real-time data processing and continuous monitoring

Explanation: The AI-based EWS's effectiveness relies on processing real-time data to detect patterns in vital signs that indicate deterioration, such as septic shock. Continuous monitoring allows for prompt alerts, enabling the medical team to intervene early and potentially save lives.

13. *Case:* A patient with diabetes and early-stage kidney disease is enrolled in a new AI-driven program at a primary care clinic. The program includes a virtual assistant that provides personalized diet advice, medication reminders, and alerts for upcoming lab tests.

    Question: What is the primary advantage of using an AI-powered virtual assistant in managing chronic conditions?

    A. Eliminating the need for follow-up appointments
    B. Improving patient adherence and engagement through tailored reminders
    C. Automating all clinical decisions related to the patient's care
    D. Replacing the role of healthcare providers entirely

    Answer: B. Improving patient adherence and engagement through tailored reminders

    Explanation: AI-powered virtual assistants improve chronic disease management by providing reminders and educational tips tailored to the patient's specific needs, leading to better adherence to treatment plans and empowering patients in self-management.

14. *Case:* A large healthcare network deploys a federated learning-based AI system across multiple hospitals to improve breast cancer detection rates. Each hospital's data remains on-site, while the AI model aggregates learnings without centralizing any patient data.

    Question: What is the main advantage of using federated learning in this setting?

    A. Reduced computational requirements for training AI models
    B. Enhanced data privacy and security by avoiding data centralization
    C. Faster individual patient diagnosis without hospital involvement
    D. Limiting model training to only the largest datasets

    Answer: B. Enhanced data privacy and security by avoiding data centralization

    Explanation: Federated learning allows hospitals to retain control of patient data, enhancing privacy and security. By aggregating learnings without centralizing data, federated learning enables collaborative model training while safeguarding sensitive information.

15. *Case:* An orthopedic clinic uses an AI tool that predicts recovery outcomes for patients undergoing knee replacement surgery based on preoperative data, such as age, weight, mobility levels, and previous health history. The tool's recommendations are used to adjust postsurgical care plans accordingly.

    Question: Which aspect of AI in healthcare is highlighted in this case?

    A. Automated surgical procedures
    B. Predictive analytics for personalized recovery planning

    C. Patient data anonymization techniques
    D. Virtual assistant interactions for surgery

Answer: B. Predictive analytics for personalized recovery planning

Explanation: Predictive analytics allows the AI tool to forecast recovery outcomes and tailor postsurgical care, enabling personalized treatment plans based on individual patient profiles, which may improve recovery times and outcomes.

16. *Case:* An oncology center implements an AI model to assist in identifying genetic markers for personalized chemotherapy regimens. The AI analyzes genetic mutations from patient samples to recommend therapies with the highest likelihood of success for each individual.

    Question: Which benefit of AI is most evident in this case?
    A. Standardized treatment plans for all cancer patients
    B. Personalized, genetics-based treatment recommendations
    C. Reduced need for human oncologists
    D. Elimination of chemotherapy side effects

    Answer: B. Personalized, genetics-based treatment recommendations

    Explanation: AI-driven analysis of genetic mutations enables personalized cancer treatments that align with each patient's unique genetic profile, increasing the likelihood of treatment efficacy and potentially minimizing unnecessary side effects.

17. *Case:* A dermatology clinic employs an AI diagnostic tool for skin cancer that can analyze images of skin lesions to classify them as benign, malignant, or requiring biopsy. The tool assists dermatologists by providing an initial assessment before they conduct a clinical examination.

    Question: What challenge might the clinic face when using this AI tool in dermatology?
    A. Inadequate patient access to AI tools
    B. Dependency on AI without adequate clinician oversight
    C. Decreased diagnostic accuracy compared to manual methods
    D. Reduced ability to analyze common skin conditions

    Answer: B. Dependency on AI without adequate clinician oversight

    Explanation: While the AI tool can provide valuable preliminary assessments, over-reliance on AI without sufficient clinician oversight could lead to errors. It is essential for clinicians to use AI as a supportive tool and not as a substitute for their expertise.

18. *Case:* A pediatric clinic integrates an AI application that analyzes developmental milestones and behavioral data to detect early signs of autism spectrum disorder (ASD). The tool flags at-risk children for further evaluation by specialists.

    Question: What is a key advantage of using AI for early autism detection in pediatric patients?
    A. Replacing the need for professional developmental assessments
    B. Identifying subtle indicators early, leading to timely intervention
    C. Avoiding any need for parental involvement
    D. Providing definitive diagnoses without further testing

    Answer: B. Identifying subtle indicators early, leading to timely intervention

Explanation: AI tools can detect subtle behavioral patterns and developmental delays that may be indicative of ASD, allowing for early intervention that can improve outcomes in children at risk.

19. *Case:* A primary care clinic uses an AI-powered predictive model that analyzes population health data to identify communities at high risk for diabetes. The clinic initiates a targeted outreach program, providing resources and education on lifestyle changes in these areas.

    Question: What AI application is demonstrated by this case?

    A. Robotic-assisted interventions
    B. Predictive analytics for population health management
    C. Autonomous patient diagnostics
    D. Natural language processing for clinic documentation

    Answer: B. Predictive analytics for population health management

    Explanation: Predictive analytics in this case identifies high-risk communities, enabling the clinic to proactively address public health concerns and promote preventive measures for diabetes management.

20. *Case:* In an ICU setting, a real-time AI system monitors multiple parameters including heart rate, oxygen saturation, and blood pressure to detect potential cases of sepsis. The AI tool alerts clinicians when abnormal patterns are identified, suggesting an elevated risk of sepsis.

    Question: What is an important consideration for clinicians when relying on this AI system in the ICU?

    A. Ensuring the system operates independently of human input
    B. Interpreting AI alerts within the broader clinical context
    C. Avoiding any form of patient interaction to reduce risk
    D. Limiting the system's access to only stable patients

    Answer: B. Interpreting AI alerts within the broader clinical context

    Explanation: While the AI system provides valuable early alerts, it is essential that clinicians interpret these alerts within the context of each patient's overall clinical status, as no AI tool can replace comprehensive clinical judgment.

21. *Case:* A pulmonology clinic introduces an AI system that analyzes patient data and environmental factors to predict asthma exacerbations. This tool integrates weather data, air quality indices, and individual patient profiles to provide early warnings for at-risk patients.

    Question: Which aspect of AI is most critical in predicting asthma exacerbations in this setting?

    A. Data integration from multiple external sources
    B. Restricting analysis to genetic predispositions
    C. Limiting the model to hospital-based data only
    D. Providing automated treatment plans

    Answer: A. Data integration from multiple external sources

    Explanation: Predicting asthma exacerbations involves incorporating data beyond the patient's health records, such as environmental factors. Effective integration of external data sources, such as weather and air quality is critical for accurate, real-time predictions.

22. *Case:* In a study on the effectiveness of AI in reducing medication errors, a hospital deployed an AI-driven prescription verification system. The system flags potential drug interactions and dosage errors before prescriptions are finalized by the physician.

    Question: What is a major limitation that clinicians should consider with this AI system?

    A. Reduced dependency on human pharmacists
    B. Potential for false positives leading to alert fatigue
    C. Requirement for patient consent for each flagged prescription
    D. Decreased efficiency in high-volume settings

    Answer: B. Potential for false positives leading to alert fatigue

    Explanation: AI-driven verification systems can sometimes generate excessive alerts, including false positives. This can lead to alert fatigue among clinicians, where they may begin ignoring or dismissing alerts, undermining the system's effectiveness.

23. *Case:* A dermatology clinic utilizes an AI-powered image recognition system to assist in diagnosing melanoma. The tool provides a probability score for malignancy based on lesion characteristics, helping dermatologists decide whether to proceed with a biopsy.

    Question: Which ethical consideration is most relevant in this scenario?

    A. Ensuring patient confidentiality during diagnosis
    B. Obtaining informed consent for AI-driven assessments
    C. Ensuring the AI completely replaces clinician judgment
    D. Limiting patient access to the AI's diagnostic score

    Answer: B. Obtaining informed consent for AI-driven assessments

    Explanation: When using AI-driven diagnostic tools, it is essential to inform patients about the role of AI in their care and obtain their consent. This transparency helps patients understand and feel comfortable with the technology used in their diagnosis.

24. *Case:* A psychiatric clinic uses an AI-driven app that monitors patients with major depressive disorder (MDD) through mood assessments and daily behavior tracking, alerting clinicians if signs of relapse are detected.

    Question: What is the primary benefit of AI in this mental health application?

    A. Automating all therapeutic decisions
    B. Allowing early detection and intervention for relapses
    C. Replacing the need for clinician involvement
    D. Limiting patient interactions to crisis situations

    Answer: B. Allowing early detection and intervention for relapses

    Explanation: AI applications in mental health can help monitor subtle changes in mood or behavior, allowing clinicians to detect potential relapses early and provide timely intervention, which is crucial in managing conditions like MDD.

25. *Case:* A hospital's intensive care unit (ICU) implements an AI tool that predicts the onset of acute respiratory distress syndrome (ARDS) based on real-time monitoring of vital signs and lab results.

    Question: Which challenge is most relevant to the implementation of this AI tool in the ICU?

    A. Ensuring clinician acceptance without skepticism
    B. Managing real-time data requirements and processing speed

C. Limiting the tool's access to only high-risk patients

D. Decreasing the overall number of ICU admissions

Answer: B. Managing real-time data requirements and processing speed

Explanation: Real-time monitoring in critical care settings requires high processing speed and accurate data integration to generate timely and actionable alerts, which can be challenging in fast-paced environments like the ICU.

26. *Case:* A primary care clinic integrates an AI model that analyzes patient records and lifestyle data to identify those at high risk for type 2 diabetes. The clinic then initiates preventive care programs for identified patients.

    Question: Which aspect of AI's role in healthcare is exemplified here?

    A. Reactive healthcare management

    B. Predictive analytics for preventive care

    C. Autonomous decision-making without oversight

    D. Reduction in overall healthcare costs

    Answer: B. Predictive analytics for preventive care

    Explanation: AI-driven predictive analytics enables early identification of individuals at risk for chronic diseases, such as diabetes, allowing healthcare providers to implement preventive measures before conditions progress.

27. *Case:* In an emergency department (ED), an AI triage system assesses incoming patients based on their symptoms and vital signs, prioritizing cases with high risk for rapid deterioration.

    Question: What is an important factor for clinicians to consider when using this AI triage system?

    A. Limiting triage decisions to senior staff only

    B. Balancing AI recommendations with clinical judgment

    C. Ensuring AI replaces all manual triage processes

    D. Applying AI triage only during off-peak hours

    Answer: B. Balancing AI recommendations with clinical judgment

    Explanation: While AI can efficiently prioritize patients, it is essential for clinicians to use their expertise to validate AI recommendations, ensuring the triage decisions align with the overall clinical picture.

28. *Case:* A nephrology clinic uses an AI model to predict patients' likelihood of progression to end-stage renal disease (ESRD) based on their lab results, lifestyle data, and genetic factors. Patients with higher risk scores receive more intensive monitoring and management.

    Question: What type of AI application is demonstrated in this scenario?

    A. Autonomous diagnosis without clinician input

    B. Predictive modeling for risk stratification

    C. Replacement of conventional nephrology tests

    D. Automated prescription of dialysis

    Answer: B. Predictive modeling for risk stratification

    Explanation: Predictive modeling enables AI to assess individual risk levels for disease progression, helping clinicians prioritize resources and tailor care to those most likely to benefit from intensive management.

29. *Case:* A general surgery department implements an AI system to assist surgeons during procedures by providing real-time anatomical guidance and identifying structures to avoid, such as nerves and blood vessels.

    Question: Which AI feature is most relevant in this surgical setting?

    A. Image recognition for real-time anatomical visualization
    B. Data aggregation across multiple surgical cases
    C. Predictive analytics for postsurgical outcomes
    D. Fully autonomous surgical procedures

    Answer: A. Image recognition for real-time anatomical visualization

    Explanation: In surgical settings, AI-driven image recognition provides real-time visual assistance, helping surgeons navigate complex anatomy with precision, which can reduce errors and improve patient outcomes.

30. *Case:* A hospital uses an AI system to monitor medication adherence in elderly patients by analyzing patterns in prescription refills and wearable data that track physical activity. Alerts are sent to healthcare providers if nonadherence is detected.

    Question: What is a primary benefit of this AI system?

    A. Reducing healthcare staff workload through automation
    B. Early detection of nonadherence and timely intervention
    C. Replacing the need for periodic medical check-ups
    D. Limiting the use of wearable data to prevent privacy issues

    Answer: B. Early detection of nonadherence and timely intervention

    Explanation: AI can identify patterns indicative of nonadherence and provide timely alerts, enabling healthcare providers to intervene and support elderly patients in maintaining their medication regimen.

31. *Case:* A large healthcare system deploys an AI-based platform to support patient referrals across departments. The AI evaluates patient records and matches them with specialists based on individual health conditions, predicted needs, and clinician availability.

    Question: What key factor should be evaluated to ensure the accuracy and fairness of this AI referral system?

    A. Availability of each specialist
    B. Inclusion of socioeconomic and demographic factors
    C. Exclusivity of referrals to high-demand specialties
    D. Limiting referrals to a single specialty

    Answer: B. Inclusion of socioeconomic and demographic factors

    Explanation: To ensure fair and accurate referrals, it is essential that the AI model accounts for demographic and socioeconomic factors, which may affect healthcare accessibility and specific patient needs, thus promoting equity in the referral process.

32. *Case:* An ICU introduces an AI model for real-time monitoring and early detection of delirium in critically-ill patients. The tool processes a combination of vital signs, medication history, and lab results to identify patients at high risk of developing delirium.

    Question: Which consideration is most important to maximize the model's effectiveness in this setting?

A. Exclusively monitoring patients with known cognitive impairments
B. Continuous data updates for real-time prediction accuracy
C. Limiting the model's application to postoperative patients only
D. Reducing alerts to avoid clinician intervention

Answer: B. Continuous data updates for real-time prediction accuracy
Explanation: Continuous data updates are crucial for the model to maintain real-time accuracy, allowing clinicians to make timely interventions for patients showing early signs of delirium.

33. *Case:* A dermatology clinic integrates an AI tool for the automatic classification of skin lesions based on images. The model provides likelihood scores for different diagnoses, but some clinicians are concerned about the accuracy of the scores in patients with darker skin tones.
   Question: What step should the clinic take to address this concern?
   A. Adjust the model to exclude patients with darker skin tones
   B. Conduct a bias audit and retrain the model with a diverse dataset
   C. Only use the model as a last-resort diagnostic tool
   D. Limit AI use to common skin conditions only

   Answer: B. Conduct a bias audit and retrain the model with a diverse dataset
   Explanation: A bias audit, followed by retraining the model on a diverse dataset, can improve the AI tool's accuracy across skin tones, ensuring it is more equitable and reliable for all patients.

34. *Case:* An endocrinology clinic uses an AI-powered platform to tailor diabetes management plans based on each patient's glucose patterns, lifestyle, and dietary habits. However, some patients struggle to follow the recommended changes due to personal constraints.
   Question: How can the clinic improve patient adherence to AI-driven recommendations?
   A. Limit the recommendations to lifestyle factors only
   B. Use an explainable AI model that aligns recommendations with patient preferences
   C. Reduce the frequency of AI-driven updates
   D. Assign each patient a universal treatment plan

   Answer: B. Use an explainable AI model that aligns recommendations with patient preferences
   Explanation: Using explainable AI can help patients understand the recommendations and how they fit into their personal lifestyles, enhancing adherence by aligning AI recommendations with patients' individual preferences and constraints.

35. *Case:* A hospital integrates an AI decision-support tool to prioritize emergency cases. The tool flags a patient's case as low priority, but the attending physician suspects a more serious condition based on clinical judgment.
   Question: What should be the primary approach to manage this discrepancy?
   A. Override the AI tool based on physician expertise
   B. Adhere strictly to the AI tool's recommendations
   C. Reassess the patient without AI input
   D. Limit physician intervention to confirmed cases only

   Answer: A. Override the AI tool based on physician expertise

Explanation: Physician expertise should take precedence over AI recommendations when clinical suspicion suggests otherwise. This approach ensures that AI serves as a supportive tool rather than replacing human judgment.

36. *Case:* A telemedicine platform powered by AI uses natural language processing (NLP) to provide real-time responses to patients' queries about chronic disease management. A patient reports confusion about conflicting AI responses on medication side effects.

    Question: How can the platform address this issue to improve patient trust?
    A. Standardize responses across all patient queries
    B. Implement stricter protocols for consistent response generation
    C. Limit responses to frequently asked questions (FAQs) only
    D. Discontinue using NLP for medication-related questions

    Answer: B. Implement stricter protocols for consistent response generation
    Explanation: To avoid inconsistencies, the platform should use standardized protocols for response generation, ensuring that patients receive clear and reliable answers that support their trust in AI.

37. *Case:* An AI tool in a primary care clinic identifies patients at high risk for hypertension based on lifestyle factors, lab results, and EHR data. However, some patients flagged as high-risk do not develop hypertension as predicted.

    Question: What might be a reason for these false positives in risk prediction?
    A. Overreliance on socioeconomic data
    B. Lack of integration with genetic factors
    C. Failure to account for recent lifestyle changes
    D. Inclusion of patient demographic data only

    Answer: C. Failure to account for recent lifestyle changes
    Explanation: If recent lifestyle improvements are not reflected in the data, the AI tool may overestimate risk. Continuous data updates or reassessment can help mitigate false positives.

38. *Case:* A tertiary care center uses an AI model to identify candidates for surgery based on disease progression data. The model sometimes prioritizes candidates with milder symptoms over those with more severe conditions.

    Question: What potential flaw might this reveal in the AI model's criteria?
    A. Overweighting of demographic data
    B. Emphasis on early intervention data rather than severity
    C. Lack of proper feature selection
    D. Bias toward certain surgical types

    Answer: B. Emphasis on early intervention data rather than severity
    Explanation: If the AI prioritizes early intervention but does not fully consider symptom severity, it may incorrectly prioritize patients, leading to flawed treatment decisions.

39. *Case:* A cardiology AI tool predicts patient risk for atrial fibrillation (AF) and suggests early interventions. A patient with a high predicted risk insists on waiting, citing a lack of symptoms.

    Question: What would be a suitable response from the clinician in this situation?

A. Explain the prediction's basis and the benefits of proactive care
B. Defer all decisions to the patient
C. Disregard the AI recommendation
D. Insist on immediate intervention

Answer: A. Explain the prediction's basis and the benefits of proactive care

Explanation: Educating the patient on how the AI prediction is made and the potential benefits of early intervention helps them make an informed choice, supporting shared decision-making.

40. *Case:* A healthcare organization deploys an AI-based workflow optimization tool for appointment scheduling, which assigns priority based on medical urgency. However, some patients with chronic conditions report delays in routine appointments.
    Question: What might improve scheduling equity in this AI system?
    A. Limiting priority scheduling to emergency cases
    B. Balancing urgent and routine care needs in the algorithm
    C. Removing routine patients from AI scheduling
    D. Standardizing appointment times regardless of urgency

    Answer: B. Balancing urgent and routine care needs in the algorithm

    Explanation: Adjusting the AI system to account for both urgent and routine needs can ensure fair access to healthcare, preventing delays in necessary ongoing care.

41. *Case:* A pediatric clinic uses an AI model to monitor vaccination compliance and predict missed appointments. The AI flags a family as likely to miss their upcoming immunization visit.
    Question: What action should the clinic consider based on this prediction?
    A. Schedule the family for an urgent appointment
    B. Send targeted reminders to the family ahead of the appointment
    C. Remove them from the immunization schedule
    D. Limit the prediction to specific immunizations

    Answer: B. Send targeted reminders to the family ahead of the appointment

    Explanation: Targeted reminders can improve attendance by addressing potential barriers proactively, supporting higher vaccination compliance without penalizing families.

42. *Case:* A surgical team uses an AI tool that analyzes computed tomography (CT) scans in real-time to highlight anatomical structures, assisting surgeons during complex operations. The AI occasionally flags structures that are not relevant to the procedure.
    Question: How can the tool be improved to reduce unnecessary flags?
    A. Narrow the focus of the AI to procedure-specific anatomy
    B. Remove certain structures from analysis
    C. Only use the AI for major surgeries
    D. Limit the AI's use to preoperative scans

    Answer: A. Narrow the focus of the AI to procedure-specific anatomy

    Explanation: Tailoring the AI to highlight only structures relevant to the specific procedure can reduce irrelevant alerts, making it more efficient and useful during surgery.

43. *Case:* A mental health clinic uses an AI-powered chatbot to support patients with anxiety by providing daily exercises and reminders. One patient reports feeling overwhelmed by the frequent notifications.

    Question: What modification might improve the patient's experience with the AI tool?

    A. Increase the frequency of notifications
    B. Allow patients to customize notification frequency
    C. Remove all reminders related to anxiety management
    D. Restrict reminders to high-severity cases

    Answer: B. Allow patients to customize notification frequency

    Explanation: Customizing notification settings allows patients to choose a frequency that suits their comfort level, enhancing engagement without causing additional stress.

44. *Case:* A radiology department uses an AI tool that classifies chest X-rays, including identifying signs of tuberculosis (TB). However, the region has a low prevalence of TB, leading to multiple false-positive alerts.

    Question: How might the AI model be optimized for this setting?

    A. Increase sensitivity for TB detection
    B. Reduce TB detection sensitivity and prioritize other conditions
    C. Limit the model's use to high-prevalence regions only
    D. Exclude TB detection from the model

    Answer: B. Reduce TB detection sensitivity and prioritize other conditions

    Explanation: Adjusting the model's sensitivity can help reduce false positives for low-prevalence conditions, making the tool more appropriate for the specific regional context.

45. *Case:* A neurologist uses an AI tool to predict the likelihood of stroke in patients with atrial fibrillation (AF). The model analyzes patient histories, lab results, and lifestyle factors to assign a stroke risk score, but recent updates make the tool's decision-making process less interpretable for the clinician.

    Question: What would be a suitable response from the healthcare team to address this issue?

    A. Limit the use of the tool only to high-risk patients
    B. Request an explainable AI model that clarifies predictions
    C. Reduce the tool's application to prevent bias
    D. Remove lifestyle factors from the model

    Answer: B. Request an explainable AI model that clarifies predictions

    Explanation: Using an explainable AI model allows clinicians to understand how risk scores are generated, which helps in making informed treatment decisions and maintaining trust in the AI tool.

46. *Case:* A hospital uses an AI-driven remote monitoring platform for elderly patients with heart failure. The platform tracks daily physical activity, heart rate, and medication adherence, alerting healthcare providers if it detects signs of decompensation.

    Question: What is a potential challenge associated with this remote monitoring system?

    A. Excessive dependency on human intervention
    B. High risk of patient data breaches

C. Increased patient disengagement due to lack of real-time updates

D. Alert fatigue for healthcare providers from frequent notifications

Answer: D. Alert fatigue for healthcare providers from frequent notifications

Explanation: Frequent alerts can overwhelm healthcare providers, leading to alert fatigue where they may ignore or miss critical notifications. Refining the alert system to prioritize urgent cases can mitigate this risk.

47. *Case:* An oncology department uses an AI model to recommend targeted cancer therapies based on genetic profiles. A patient with limited financial resources expresses concerns about the costs associated with the recommended treatment.

    Question: How should the healthcare team address this concern?

    A. Suggest a different, less effective treatment

    B. Seek support from financial assistance programs for treatment costs

    C. Disregard the AI recommendation to avoid financial strain

    D. Delay treatment until finances are resolved

    Answer: B. Seek support from financial assistance programs for treatment costs

    Explanation: The healthcare team should help the patient access financial assistance to afford the recommended targeted therapy, ensuring that the AI-driven recommendation aligns with both medical and financial feasibility.

48. *Case:* A pediatric hospital employs an AI tool to detect signs of childhood developmental delays through natural language processing of interactions and behavioral data from wearable devices.

    Question: What should be prioritized to ensure the ethical use of this AI tool in children?

    A. Regular updates to improve algorithm speed

    B. Parental consent and transparency regarding data usage

    C. Limiting data collection to ensure lower costs

    D. Reducing clinician involvement in diagnosis

    Answer: B. Parental consent and transparency regarding data usage

    Explanation: Ensuring parental consent and transparency about data collection and use are crucial for ethical AI applications involving minors, as these practices maintain trust and protect children's privacy rights.

49. *Case:* A rural clinic uses an AI-based triage system to assist in diagnosing common conditions due to limited access to specialists. However, some patients report discomfort with relying solely on AI for medical decisions.

    Question: What adjustment could help address patient concerns in this setting?

    A. Provide additional human oversight and communication about AI's role

    B. Reduce the AI's application scope to only emergency cases

    C. Limit the AI system to lower-risk patients

    D. Exclude specific demographics from AI diagnosis

    Answer: A. Provide additional human oversight and communication about AI's role

    Explanation: Enhancing human oversight and explaining that AI supports, rather than replaces, clinical decision-making can alleviate patient concerns, fostering trust and acceptance of AI in medical triage.

50. *Case:* A mental health provider uses an AI chatbot to provide 24/7 support for patients with anxiety, offering exercises and coping mechanisms. A patient becomes overly dependent on the chatbot, reducing engagement in face-to-face therapy sessions.

    Question: What modification could improve this patient's engagement in traditional therapy?

    A. Discontinue chatbot access altogether
    B. Encourage balanced use of AI and in-person therapy
    C. Restrict chatbot interaction to emergency support only
    D. Increase chatbot's frequency of sessions to replace therapy

    Answer: B. Encourage balanced use of AI and in-person therapy

    Explanation: Educating the patient on the value of balancing chatbot use with in-person therapy can enhance engagement in traditional treatment, preventing over-reliance on AI alone for mental health management.

51. *Case:* A hospital uses an AI system to prioritize patients for liver transplant lists based on factors, such as organ compatibility, urgency, and waiting time. Some patients and families raise ethical concerns about transparency in AI-driven decision-making.

    Question: What would be an appropriate response from the healthcare organization?

    A. Remove AI's role in the transplant decision-making process
    B. Increase transparency by explaining how AI criteria impact decisions
    C. Limit AI's use to nonurgent transplant cases
    D. Allow patients to opt out of AI-based prioritization

    Answer: B. Increase transparency by explaining how AI criteria impact decisions

    Explanation: Explaining the AI's role in prioritizing transplants and clarifying how its criteria align with clinical guidelines can address ethical concerns and build trust in AI-based decision-making.

52. *Case:* An orthopedic clinic uses an AI model to predict recovery times for patients undergoing knee replacement surgery, based on factors, such as age, weight, and comorbidities. A younger, healthy patient receives a longer predicted recovery time than expected.

    Question: What should the clinician consider before discussing this prediction with the patient?

    A. The possibility of bias in the AI model's training data
    B. Adjusting the recovery prediction manually
    C. Limiting AI use to patients over a certain age
    D. Using the AI only for high-risk patients

    Answer: A. The possibility of bias in the AI model's training data

    Explanation: Before presenting a recovery time prediction, the clinician should consider that the AI model may be biased based on training data and verify that predictions align with expected norms for a patient with the individual's profile.

53. *Case:* A cardiology AI tool evaluates lifestyle data from wearable devices to recommend lifestyle modifications for patients with hypertension. A patient receives suggestions to increase exercise, which conflicts with their orthopedic limitations.

    Question: How should the healthcare provider address this AI recommendation?

    A. Adhere strictly to the AI recommendation
    B. Adjust the recommendation based on the patient's physical limitations
    C. Instruct the patient to ignore AI's lifestyle advice
    D. Reduce AI access to physical activity data

    Answer: B. Adjust the recommendation based on the patient's physical limitations
    Explanation: The healthcare provider should modify the AI recommendation to align with the patient's orthopedic constraints, ensuring lifestyle advice is realistic and personalized to their specific needs.

54. *Case:* A hospital system implements an AI-based patient scheduling tool that attempts to reduce wait times by optimizing appointment slots based on patient history and needs. However, some patients with complex conditions feel rushed in shorter appointments.

    Question: What adjustment might improve the system's scheduling fairness?

    A. Exclude complex cases from AI scheduling
    B. Allow flexibility in appointment length for patients with complex needs
    C. Standardize all appointments to the shortest duration
    D. Use AI for scheduling follow-up visits only

    Answer: B. Allow flexibility in appointment length for patients with complex needs
    Explanation: Providing flexibility in appointment durations based on patient complexity can help accommodate those with more extensive needs, ensuring equitable access to care.

55. *Case:* An AI-powered imaging tool is used in an oncology clinic to assess tumor progression from magnetic resonance imaging (MRI) scans. The AI flags rapid progression, but the oncologist suspects it may be a false positive due to imaging artifacts.

    Question: What should the oncologist do in response to the AI's flag?

    A. Proceed with aggressive treatment without further testing
    B. Confirm the AI's findings with additional imaging or testing
    C. Ignore the AI's recommendation altogether
    D. Rely on the AI's flag as the final diagnosis

    Answer: B. Confirm the AI's findings with additional imaging or testing
    Explanation: Verifying AI findings with further imaging ensures that decisions are based on accurate information, especially when there is potential for false positives due to imaging artifacts.

Index

N

O

P

EU GSPR Authorised Reprsentative
Logos Europe, 9 rue Nicolas Poussin
1700, La Rochelle, France
Phone: +33 (0) 6 67 93 73 78
E-mail: contact@logoseurope.eu

www.ingramcontent.com/pod-product-compliance
Ingram Content Group UK Ltd.
Pitfield, Milton Keynes, MK11 3LW, UK
UKHW051940150726
7214IPUK00020B/358